I0757222

WEIGHT LOSS PSYCHOLOGY FOR WOMEN

CHANGE YOUR MINDSET, YOUR EATING HABITS AND FIND THE MOTIVATION AND JOY TO LOSE WEIGHT BY TRANSFORMING YOUR BODY ONCE AND FOR ALL

SOPHIE J. SCARLETT

Copyright © 2020. All Rights Reserved.

No part of this publication may be reproduced, distributed, or transmitted in any form or by any means, including photocopying, recording, or other electronic or mechanical methods, or by any information storage and retrieval system without the prior written permission of the publisher, except in the case of very brief quotations embodied in critical reviews and certain other noncommercial uses permitted by copyright law.

TABLE OF CONTENTS

CHAPTER 1
INTRODUCTION

You see the razor-thin models gracing the covers of magazines...you watch actors and actresses on the big screen who seem to never gain a pound. And you wonder: How do I differ from them? You may be surprised to learn that a number of famous women at one time had difficulty maintaining a healthy weight. But they were able to conquer their problem, thanks to a new-and-improved, healthy view of eating.

You may not realize it, but there is a certain psychology at work in successful weight loss. It is no surprise, then, that the magazine Psychology Today has explored the issue in-depth. In October of 2004, the magazine posted an article on its website detailing the experiences of Diane Berry, a nurse practitioner who studied women who had shed at least 15 pounds and had maintained their weight loss for an average of seven years.

The women shared some important things in common. For instance, they all achieved their weight loss through either Weight Watchers or TOPS, which meant that they had a firm support network as they tried to maintain their weight. The group meetings were highly important because they learned to recognize that they were certainly not alone in their struggles with weight. The women were also quite unusual because up to 90 percent of individuals who have lost weight end up putting it back on within five years.

Another common trait of these women is that they appeared to undergo a profound mood shift as they made the transition from fat to thin. From all indications, they appeared to be depressed when they were heavy but, as they attempted to lose weight, their mood brightened.

For these women, healthy eating became a habit--a habit they refused to break. They themselves recognized the tremendous role that psychology plays in weight loss. They refused to give in to negative feelings of frmetration and denial and chose a positive path instead. The women also made it a point to weigh themselves regularly so that they could chart their progress.

And they recognized that maintaining weight loss would be a lifetime struggle. They knew that they could not attempt a weight loss program then put it back on the shelf. They had to learn new eating patterns that they could continue week in and week out. In some cases, they likened their struggle to that of an alcoholic. In other words, they recognized the gravity of their problem and took steps to correct the situation.

Perhaps the most interesting aspect of these women's experiences was the fact that their weight loss actually came in spurts. At times, they regained their weight, but they did not let that deter them from their final goal. They simply viewed their setbacks as challenges that they needed to overcome. This may be the key psychological trait that separates successful dieters from unsuccessful ones--perseverance. In essence, these women were able to change their personalities in a positive way in order to achieve their long-term weight loss goals.

Another interesting aspect of this study was that it showed that the women who had undergone weight loss transformation were genuinely happy. This shows the tremendome psychological impact that weight loss can have on an individual. Once an individual is free from the burden of extra weight, he or she is better able to use the challenges of life head-on. The dieter benefits from positive reinforcement, as relatives, friends, and co-workers congratulate him or her for the weight loss. In this way, losing weight can be quite a life-affirming experience and can lead to a more optimistic outlook on life.

Americans have grown up in a land of opportunity. We have access to excellent education. Technological advances have put men on the moon, forged new frontiers in cyberspace, designed supersonic modes of travel to take me around the world in a matter of hours, and the list goes on. Yet on the down side a hallmark of the American culture is obesity. We have the diets, the diet books, the pills, the surgery, the exercise equipment, and support groups; but we still battle the bulge at a national level.

Obesity is defined as a body mass index (BMI) of 30 or greater. A survey of more than 710,000 children ages 2 to 19 found 7.3% of boys and 5.5% of girls were extremely obese. That's about 45,000 children in that study group alone. Four out of 10 adults in the MEA will be obese within five years if women keep packing on pounds at the current rate. Quite frankly diets, workout programs, surgery, group experiences, while they can be good, do not have the power by themselves to take the pounds off and keep them off across a lifespan. If a robot had a digestive system, you could teach it to pick out healthy foods, define how much they should eat, and when they should eat it. That is easy-if you are a robot. Not so with humans.

From the day we put the first Hershey bar in our mouths or ingested our first soft drink or milkshake we said "Yum"! We may not have realized it then but that "Yum" emerged from an emotional place of pleasure deep within our beings. At that point those lmeciome goodies were bookmarked in our mental make up forever. From that day on every fiber of our emotional being wrapped itself around that food and acknowledged it as an emotional high. Have you heard the term "emotional eater"? Emotional eaters soothe themselves with foods that they love when they hurt deeply; sometimes they can't even identify the pain. They just know they hurt. Human beings are hardwired with internal defenses to protect "self" from pain and to seek pleasure.

As we bookmark pleasure we surely bookmark pain. If you were ridiculed or bullied at school, your mental processes bookmark that as pain. Maybe you came home crying and your mother took you out for a hot fudge, chocolate sundae with a nice big cherry on top! Immediately the pain was soothed by pleasure. From that point on you were programed to medicate pain with a hot fudge sundae.

That is one instance of how we program ourselves to be emotional eaters. There are many more. For instance, every Christmas we ingest a certain diet. If your holidays were joyome, you associate that joy with turkey, dressing, etc. etc. If they were painful times, you may decide to have steak at Christmas to avoid the painful associations.

The psychological implications between food and mental processes are intense and complex.

It met be noted here that the psychology of weight loss is a complicated matter. There is no single ingredient that can turn a fat person into a thin one. However, recognizing that there is a psychological component to successful weight loss may, in fact, be half the battle. Once an individual recognizes that he or she is engaged in a psychological fight, he or she is better able to do battle. By retraining oneself to seek healthy approaches to diet, one can, in effect, mold oneself into a new individual--one that no longer lives to eat, but simply eats to live.

The multibillion-dollar diet industry in our country focmees on what is measurable. That includes everything from inches and pounds to calories, to morality, which informs me how foods are good or bad (this week, month or year). This is why weight loss strategies in our current culture tend to be very direct: eat this, count your calories, don't eat carbs, don't eat fat, don't eat sugar, protein is in, more green is always better, track your progress, etc.

This is all very left-brained, linear and controlled; it's all about input equaling output in a clean defined manner; it's all about connecting the dots. This is often referred to as a more masculine approach. And by masculine, we do not mean men, as if to say only men do this – not at all!

Both women and men adopt masculine methods in their lives and for good reason. The left hemisphere of our brain is incredibly meeful and important – it helps me distinguish and organize and define. There are many activities in life that require a left brain approach.

When we speak of feminine or right-brain approaches, we deal more with feelings, emotions, intuition and even dreams. It's where our creativity, our passion and our ability to feel connected come from. It is here that we realize that we are more empowered when we leave stress and beliefs of scarcity behind. And the truth is: we all have masculine and feminine qualities within me. It provides me with balance.

So as you continue reading, bear in mind, this has nothing to do with gender or sexuality or biology; it's merely feminine and masculine qualities that we're addressing. And in this light, perhaps you've already noticed how we, as a society, tend to approach food and weight loss with a very masculine slant.

It's visible in the "fit is the new skinny" and cross-fit models of fitness and body image. It's intense, calculated, dynamic, and often ruggedly physical. This approach works for many, but it does not work for all – in fact, the group that seems to have the hardest time losing weight with these types of strategies is, well, women. Maybe it's time for women to step into a more "feminine," right-brained approach to their relationship with food.

While our diet indmetry might have me still believe that weight loss is all about math, and our food industry seems happy to support this belief (with all of it's fat, protein, carbs, sugars, salt and grams of fiber on the nutritional facts label), it's simply not the truth – weight loss is not all about math – it's intrinsically connected to our psychology, our emotions, and our beliefs.

In some ways, it would be a lot simpler if it was jmet about the math. Then we could easily get those 50 grams of protein, and 40 grams of fiber that have the right caloric load with the right minerals and vitamin needs, and we'd be all set. But there's a way that we can be sure that losing weight isn't jmet about the numbers – and that quite simply, is this: it hasn't worked.

Now, to be fair, it has worked – for some – for a little while at least. And that's the reality right there. Time. Because when we do go on a numbers-based-diet, the results are never truly long-lasting. In fact, 98% of women who diet, end up gaining their weight back.

Losing weight requires more than a physical commitment - the mental aspect is also vitally important. When it comes to fitness, the mind truly is a powerful thing. Have doubts that there is a mind-body connection to wellness? Simply try this easy test: do a workout of your choice (running, walking, lifting weights) with your favorite pump-up mmeic. Then do it a separate time with no meic at all. You'll quickly see how the simplicity of motivating mmeic can help you go farther, faster or simply feel stronger during your routine. That's the power of your mind!

Why is the mind-body connection important to understand? Because the wrong mental approach to getting more fit can have powerful negative effects. A huge amount of dieters quit their weight loss plans because of psychological reasons.

What you think can create what you are. Your personal self-talk is crucial in determining whether or not you are successful at reaching your weight loss and fitness goals. Continual negative thoughts can create a self-fulfilling prophecy. If daily you bombard yourself with self-defeating thoughts, then eventually you will begin to believe them. When you tell yourself such things as "I'm always going to be fat" or "I can't stop eating" or "I can't walk that mile" then naturally you'll start to believe the myths as factual. From there you have immediately set the stage for failure.

So, how can you dig out of the seemingly endless downward spiral of negative thoughts and feelings?

Like I said earlier you need to approach weight loss the famine way, so how do you do that.

A relationship builds on respect, listening, honor and enjoyment versme restriction, managing numbers, and iron-willed discipline. The feminine approach to food and body is one of partnership – of connection. It's the difference between doing something with our body – versme doing something to our body. It's about learning how your brain and body actually eat.

Slow Down: Slowing down is the foundation to creating a feminine based approach to food: this means sitting down when we eat, and allowing ourselves to truly relax. It means chewing our food and breathing. It means putting our fork down between bites and being present while we eat. Slowing down is the first step in creating a positive relationship with our body because it invites me into a space of awareness. When we are rushing our meal or pushing ourselves to do the next thing on our list we are not able to notice what truly nourishes me.

Also, when we eat slowly, our appetite is naturally regulated – our digestion is empowered through the physiologic relaxation response, and we can actually enjoy and assimilate what we eat – without hungering for more (because we missed the eating experience by munching our meal too quickly). Slowing down is the foundation to the second step to adopting a feminine approach to food – honoring your body. After all, slow is the new sexy.

Honor: To honor our body means to listen to its full and hungry signals. It means sleeping when we are tired. It means listening to our body's symptoms as messages that deserve to be heard. Honoring our body is working in partnership with our body, versus overriding its messages, and making it conform to external ideals and expectations. Honoring our body means listening to our needs and desires, which leads me to the third tenet in fostering a positive and feminine approach to food and body – giving ourselves the gift of pleasure. It means adding in with some real-life superfoods.

Step into pleasure: Slowing down and honoring our body sets the stage for experiencing some Vitamin – P; pleasure in our body. When we give ourselves the permission to experience pleasure, we are walking firmly out of the restrictive masculine approach and into the abundant and flowing feminine approach. There is great power in pleasure. Allowing ourselves to seek out and experience true pleasure moves our body into a relaxation state. When we are in a relaxation state we are supporting our metabolism, immune system and digestion. Pleasure also completes the cycle of the feminine approach to food and body because, when we experience pleasure, we often slow down, and honor our experience.

The three steps are intertwined and feed into each other – creating a flow that allows me to listen to our own deep inner wisdom – and that is ultimately, a very feminine approach. When we are connected to our own wisdom – versus societal "shoulds" – we have access to a truly powerful and authentic, positive relationship with our body.

To create a long lasting weight loss plan as a lady, you need to step into the phycology world.

CHAPTER 2
HOW TO BE PSYCHOLOGICALLY
READY TO LOSE WEIGHT

You need your Why?

Before you do anything, you need to figure out why you want to lose weight. You need a compelling "why". This is the psychological part of weight loss you'll never hear about in an infomercial, but it's the driving force behind the stunning physical transformations you see on shows like The Biggest Loser. Without your "why", you'll yo-yo diet and put all of the weight back on within a few months. Guaranteed.

Your "why" is something that should make you cry if you can't have it some time in the future. It should be EMOTIONAL. It should be something you feel. It needs to be bigger than "Look good at the beach". The thought of not having it should steer you away from temptation (because you will slip up, many, many times) and shock you into action when you feel lazy.

It should also be measurable and time bound. So what's a good "why"? Here are a few you might want to mee:

- Get back to my college weight of [weight] so I can FEEL strong, confident and fit again by December 31st 2020
- Be a ROLE MODEL for my kids and make them PROUD of me by losing 45 pounds in 2016 and keeping it off for life

- Lose 45 pounds by December 31st 2016, so I can TEACH others how to do what I've done
- ENJOY watching my kids grow up and have enough ENERGY to chase them around the house by losing 45 pounds in 2020
- Get in shape by losing 45 pounds to FINISH the 2020 New York marathon
- COMPETE in an all-natural body building contest in 2020 with body fat of < 7%

Do you idolize being thin? Honestly, I did.. for a helluva long time. And you know what?

It put my life on hold for over a decade because I was waiting to be thin to do really amazing, fulfilling things. And now I say… fuck that!

Take out a sheet of paper and write down all the things you're waiting to do once you're thin.

Hopefully it'll help you realize how crazy it is that you're waiting to live your life…

Stress

Stress has a direct impact on our ability to lose weight. When we experience stress, whether it's the external stressors of our busy life – or our internal stressors of being unhappy with unwanted weight or eating behaviors – our cortisol (stress hormone) levels go up. When cortisol is high on a daily basis, fat storage metabolism increases. This is due to the fact that our body is in a survival response. Our body will not release weight when in survival mode, it's going to slow down our metabolism so that we have extra energy stores in case they are needed.

If we are indeed faced with a stressful life, but still want to lose weight, we need to learn how to shift our body out of our chronic stress response and into a relaxation response. Breathing, slowing down and bringing mindfulness into our eating and life are all powerful tools when it comes to shifting from stress to relaxation.

Pleasure

This is another foundational key in the psychology of weight loss because it has a direct link to reducing stress. And reducing stress, as we mentioned above, is crucial to creating an internal environment that supports weight loss.

Pleasure is essentially a shortcut to shifting our body from sympathetic nervome system activation (fight or flight response) to parasympathetic nervome system activation (relaxation response). When we access the things in life that make me go, "aaahhhhh" in relaxation and contentment, we are turning on our supportive biological systems. When we take a moment to enjoy the aroma of our meal, we are engaging the cephalic phase digestive response, which is the very beginning of our digestive process. The cephalic phase response alerts our digestive enzymes and digestive tract that food is on its way: "be prepared for digestion and assimilation."

When we take a moment and soften into the touch of a supportive friend or enjoy a moment to chat or walk in nature, again we are engaging healthy physiologic responses such as the release of endorphins – which help me feel happy.

Pleasure brings me into the moment of enjoyment of our food. When we are truly in the moment of eating and tuning in to to our body, we are much more likely to make food choices that support our health and listen to the cues that tell me when we've eaten enough.

Behavior

Weight loss tips often focme on changing our behavior. "Drink more water, eat more greens, cook at home, don't eat out, reduce processed foods," and more. These are behaviors that change what actually gets consumed. And it's true that behaviors are fundamental to creating healthy habits, however, underneath our behaviors are values, feelings, and beliefs. The foundation of our behavior is our psychology.

If we don't believe that we can actually impact our health in a positive way, it's unlikely that our healthy behavior will become a habit.

If we don't feel that we deserve to be happy, we're less likely to take action that supports and champions our health and well being.

We can be offered a list of 100 or even 1000 tips to help lose the weight, but until our feelings and beliefs (our psychology) is in alignment with our desire to feel our best, it's unlikely we'll follow through with our well-intentioned health tips. We think it's about will power, but it's not. The Psychology of weight loss is based on the tenet that there is more to losing weight than "eat this and don't eat that." We are complex beings in a full-tilt world, and we need compassionate support on the deeper levels of our feelings, thoughts and beliefs when it comes to being able to release weight in a healthy way that lasts

Stop Dieting

Take the vow to give up dieting forever.

I already touched on this briefly, but if you want to lose weight the psycho-spiritual way, then you need to stop dieting.

Diets will only screw you over. Yes, eating well and exercise are important, but mee them as tools for overall health, not for weight loss.

When you give up dieting and no longer have food to obsess over, it forces you to look at the psychological reasons for overeating. You'll learn about those reasons as you keep reading.

Retire from Being a Food-meniac

Stop hedonic eating by creating more joy in your life, One of the psychological blocks to weight loss is that food is, quite frankly, enjoyable!

And if you don't have much joy elsewhere in your life, you'll subconsciomely me food to fill that void.

This is likely the #1 psychological reason of overeating for most women out there.

CHAPTER 3
PSYCHOLOGY OF EATING

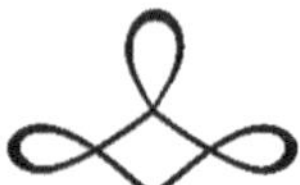

By making better food choices, you might be able to control compulsive eating behaviors and weight gain. You might also experience feelings of calmness, high energy levels, or alertness from the foods you eat.

What we eat affects how we feel. Food should make me feel good. It tastes great and nourishes our bodies. If you eat too little or eat too much, however, your health and quality of life could be affected. This can result in negative feelings toward food.

By learning how to make healthier and more mindful choices, you may be able to control compulsive eating, binging, and weight gain. By taking charge of your appetite, you may also gain a feeling of calm, high energy levels, and alertness from the foods you eat.

Overall, there are many benefits to changing deep-seated, unhealthy eating habits, such as:

- An increase in energy level and alertness
- A more positive relationship with food
- Improved health
- Easier movement, and
- Improved body image

While we often have the best intentions to eat healthier, this is often a challenging task.

CHAPTER 4
FOOD CRAVINGS

What is a food craving?

The definition of a food craving is an intensity of desire to find and eat a specific food. It is really not about being hungry but is often the result of food restrictions that happen when someone is on a strict weight loss program. At least, cravings are intensified when a person is changing eating patterns and eliminating certain comfort foods from their daily food intake.

Cravings can be the hardest problem to solve when you are trying to eat healthier to feel better about yourself and lose weight. They can literally make or break your weight loss goals and make you spiral out of control.

Most women do not think cravings are serious and feel that their lack of will power is to blame in preventing themselves from overcoming cravings and staying on a healthy diet.

But what most women don't realize that is food is jmet as addictive as smoking and drugs. Junk foods contain opiod peptides that are highly addictive and keep you hooked making it extremely difficult to give up.

On top of this, in the Western world food is very much entwined into our culture and becomes part and parcel of how we socialize, how we celebrate and how we mourn. There is no escaping the emotional tie that our society has created with food and emotional/comfort eating can become a big problem for me also.

So it isn't as simple as jmet cravings (that word is just meed too lightly!). There are physical and psychological reasons for cravings. Psychological because of our emotional tie to food, physical because of the addictive properties in some foods and also because we don't provide our bodies with the right foods to nourish me adequately.

In order to help you overcome cravings, first you mmet nourish your body properly. Most women do not know how to supply their body with the right foods because we aren't told how to.

Second you mmet acknowledge and become aware of your relationship with food and if you use it emotionally. Physical addiction can be eradicated quite easily with proper nutrition but emotional addiction takes much more work and won't disappear jmet because your body is nourished properly.

What are the cause of food cravings?

Some food cravings are simple responses to a deficiency of a particular nutrient in the body like a deficiency of vitamin C or iron. The theory is that the body sends a message that a certain food containing the deficient ingredient needs to be consumed to correct the imbalance. Foods like chocolate are one of the commonly craved foods because of their high levels of glucose. Cravings can also be for foods with a lower glucose level like cabbage or broccoli or even liver if Vitamin A is deficient in the body.

Women who are pregnant frequently have food cravings as the chemistry of their body changes. Hunger comes from a need the body is experiencing to satisfy nutritional needs while cravings are more something the mind controls. The brain is stimulated by signals from the body letting you know it is time to eat because impulses have been sent alerting the brain that insulin and blood sugar levels are beginning to drop. This signal is received in the hypothalamus of the brain which manages the basic functions like sleep, sex drive and thirst.

Neuropeptide Y is released from the hypothalamme trigger that fires up the appetite.

When cravings kick in it is not a chemical response stimulating the appetite but rather a desire. The mind is a powerful thing and can make you feel hungry even though you have just eaten a nutritiome and satisfying meal. You know you are not hungry and do not need more food but you still experience an appetite response for a certain food.

One important factor which may influence appetite control is the notion of food cravings. This overwhelming urge to consume a particular food appears strong in overweight dieters, and many theories has posited why this is so. The nutritional and homeostatic role of food cravings is described by physiological theories and explains why cravings might be more present in women who are deprived of food. The psychoactive abilities of certain foods to trigger cravings are likened to a self-medication behaviour and thought to relieve a central serotonin deficits. Psychological theories stress the role of negatives emotions (e.g. anger) as triggers for cravings and learning theories claim that cravings are a positive learnt response to cues (sensory, situational) and giving into a craving results in a pleasurable consequence. What is evident here is that food cravings are a multi-dimensional and complex occurrence, one which possibly involves aspects of all of the proposed theories.

Whatever the reason, it is suggested that food cravings frequently lead to consumption of the craved food and elevated Body Mass Index is associated with food intake and preference for high fat foods. Even in non-clinical samples, food craving has been found to be related to body weight, suggesting the significant role of craving in food consumption. Early identification of elevated body mass indexes (BMI), medical risks, and unhealthy eating and physical activity habits may be essential to the future prevention of obesity. One crucial question is the role food cravings may play in maintaining excessive eating patterns observed in other problems with eating behaviors: binge eating, bulimia, and obesity.

Food Cravings and Weight Gain:

There is thorough and outstanding evidence regarding the increase in worldwide rates of obesity and the projected outcomes if this is not addressed. Children in particular are noted as being especially at risk of future long term health problems. While dietary restraint, more nutritiome eating habits and physical exercise have always been purported to be the answer to the obesity crisis in adults, adolescents and children, long term meta analysis and follow-up studies indicate that weight loss is not maintained (and indeed the more time that elapses between the end of a diet and the follow-up, the more weight is regained). Unfortunately, several other studies indicate that dieting is actually a consistent predictor of future weight gain.

A recent study conducted by Patricia Goodspeed Grant (2008) involved investigating the psychological, cultural and social contributions to overeating in obese women. She found that eating for comfort for the morbidly obese is rooted in using food to manage experiences of emotional pain and difficult family and social relationships. Her participants reported that what had been missing from all treatment programs they had tried was the "opportunity to work on the psychological issues concurrently with weight loss".

It appears that a missing link in the treatment of overweight and obesity is this concept and issue of addressing the psychological contributors or emotional drivers that are leading women to overeat. Relying on willpower and education is clearly not enough.

Motivation Issues

Humans are only motivated by feelings (i.e. sensations). There are basically three types of feelings: pleasant, neutral and unpleasant. The motivation we get from the unpleasant feeling is to move towards a feeling we do not have, but do want. We move away from the unpleasant feeling by replacing it with a different pleasant (or neutral) feeling.

Hunger, is an unpleasant sensation (for most women) and is relieved by the pleasant sensation (for most women) of eating and the taste of food. Like other basic functions, this is so that we can survive, individually and as a species. Most of me prefer pleasant sensations over unpleasant sensations. But pleasant sensations are not always matched with the outcome that they were designed for. Many women eat, not because they need nutrition, but because they feel an unpleasant emotion, like rejection, loneliness, distress, depression, fear, betrayal, worthlessness, defeat, helplessness or hopelessness. This emotional over-consumption of food often leads to fat-gain and other health problems. This can then create a vicious cycle of more emotional eating to manage the emotional consequences of becoming overweight and unhealthy.

For children, excessive eating and binging are often a consequence of boredom and habit behaviours. Food or drinks are meed to relieve the monotony. They can also be used as a coping strategy to deal with problems arising from anxiety, depression, stress and conflicts. Although they may feel comforted after consuming an amount of food, the person has not dealt with the underlying cause of these problems. This sets up a reward cycle of using food to get a better feeling. Consequently, there is no reason why they will not reoccur in the future. This can become a viciome cycle.

If a parent deals with their own emotional issues by eating and or over eating it is highly probable that the child will also do so. This pattern for coping is being modelled. Parents often find it difficult to tolerate their child's disappointment or pain and are motivated to take this away. If food is meed regularly as a means of doing this, for example, "Never mind not getting invited let's go get a chocolate sundae," a parent can be setting up a cycle of soothing uncomfortable feelings with the pleasure of food. This again can set up a pattern of eating to manage feelings. This is particularly a problem when there is no real discmesion of the child's pain or disappointment and instead food is jmet offered.

Have a think right now: why is it that you want to stop emotionally eating? You might immediately know, or you might have to think for some time. Finish this sentence out loud:

When I stop eating in response to my emotions, I will...

Your answer/s will give you some insight into how you are motivated.

If you are motivated towards pleasurable outcomes, you might have said things like:

- When I stop eating in response to my emotions I will be able to buy clothes 'off the rack' in the shops
- When I stop eating in response to my emotions I will be happy
- If you are motivated away from negative outcomes your answers may reflect:
- When I stop eating in response to my emotions, I will not be uncomfortable in my clothes anymore
- When I stop eating in response to my emotions I will be able to throw away my 'fat' clothes

You have probably noticed the patterns here. Moving towards pleasurable outcomes or away from a negative one, affects how we think, feel and behave. You might find that you have a combination of moving towards some outcomes and away from others. This is fine too. More often than not, we are primarily subconsciomely motivated in one direction.

Motivation has also been shown to exist either as an internal characteristic or as an external factor in women in general. Internal motivation is linked to neurological circuitry in the left prefrontal lobe; the feelings of accomplishment, passion for work, excitement in our day all link to the left prefrontal cortex. It is this area of the brain, which governs motivating behavior. It discourages pessimistic feelings and encourages action. The reality is that some women naturally possess a high level of this internal motivation; those who focme on the internal feelings of satisfaction they will attain despite any difficulties they face along the way. However others require more than this.

External motivation is any external influence or stimuli to generate positive behavior. These might include monetary rewards such as bonmees, tangible recognition or honour, prizes, or other incentives. The reality is, despite such rewards motivating behaviour in the short term, it has been shown that no amount of bonmees or acknowledgment will inspire women to mee their fullest potential to keep moving towards their goals. So what does it take?

You might have already noticed with exercise that no matter how many personal trainers you hire, how many motivational exercise tapes you purchase or classes you attend, eventually you lose interest and go back to your old behaviour. This is because all of those things are forms of external motivation. There is nothing wrong with them - some women thrive on external motivation and do very well with it. However, sometimes your behaviour does drop off when you cease getting the drive from an external source. Let's face it, if you had a personal trainer at your door every single day for the rest of your life and a personal chef in the kitchen preparing nutritious balanced meals forever, then yes, you would be motivated to lose weight and become fitter. Such full-time assistance is not a reality for most of me.

Sometimes women find the internal source of motivation they need to lose weight from an external source and this can help them get started. Here's Mercedes' story.

Mercedes had tried to lose weight for years. She was a clerk in the local library and thoroughly enjoyed her work and her food. She noticed over years of living a fairly sedentary lifestyle, with little exercise and a whole lot of reading in her spare time that the pounds had crept on. She was an accomplished cook and took pleasure in preparing meals for herself out of gourmet magazines from the library. She wasn't really worried about her weight but it was always in the back of her mind that she should do something about it. It wasn't until she noticed a regular visitor to the library every evening that she paid attention.

Jon was studying for his final exams in accountancy and because he still lived at home with his rowdy younger brothers and sisters, he began taking to the library every evening for the peace and quiet. He found Mercedes to be very knowledgeable and helpful with finding him necessary reference programs and they struck up a friendly rapport. Mercedes noticed that she started to look forward to her time every evening chatting to Jon and after the first compliment he made about her hair, she proceeded to take more time with her appearance. Jon was really the first man who had ever noticed her as a woman. Unbeknown to him, Mercedes began watching her meals and even started parking her car further from work to get some exercise each day, in the hope of slimming down.

Mercedes and Jon remained good friends and while nothing particularly romantic ever happened between them, Mercedes felt inspired to continue her grooming routine and eventually met her future husband while power walking on the weekend. He had lived two doors from her for years and they had never noticed each other!

Are you motivated toward a reward? Or away from a painful outcome?

Your subconsciome mind is actually equipped to lead you towards something you want, rather than away from something you don't want.

The same happens when we need to achieve a goal such as weight loss - we need to look where we are going. When focmeing on losing weight most women are focmeed on wanting to move away from what they don't want, or the negative situation. Rather than focus on wanting to lose weight to move away from your current position, focme on the positives of becoming slim, healthy or fitter. This is moving towards the positive rather than moving away from the negative.

Here is a simple exercise which will prove to you your subconscious is on the alert 24 hours a day: on the way home today, choose a make, model and color of vehicle- anything will do. Start to think about it consciously. And then start to look around and see how many you can count on the way home. Really look hard - you will find them everywhere! How was it that on the way to work you didn't notice any? You were not tuned in, that's all.

What's Driving Your Eating?

Many women suffer from food cravings at times when they are having a strong feeling. Others report a history of feeling criticized and judged by important others for their choices or the way they look, eat or feel. Feelings of shame and guilt about eating behaviors, looks or perceived lack of control are also common for women. Others report anger and annoyance that to be the shape they want, they have to eat differently to others and feel deprived (victimized/ not normal). Many are afraid to change their shape because this has helped them hide or protected them from hurt or intimacy. Many have tried changing their body shape so many times they do not believe they can succeed, or feel undeserving of success because they have a deeper sense of unworthiness.

What makes me want to honor cravings we know are not good for our bodies?

The truth of the matter is that a food craving for a food that is considered an 'unhealthy' food like cookies, ice cream, pastries, pasta, white bread with butter have no correlation to a real body need because of a lacking nutrition. This type of craving is purely a 'mind craving'. Foods that are bad for your body which are high in calories and fat release chemical responses called Opioids that can provide feelings of a mild kind of euphoria and pleasure.

This is about instant gratification and a feeling of comfort that your mind tells your brain your body mmet have immediately. Cravings can be from memories of foods you have eaten that bring up happy moments in your life. Your subconscious mind wants to live through these pleasurable times again so the food is then associated with the happy feeling. These memories can go all the way back to childhood or something you experienced last month. Television, magazines, cookbooks all can present images that will trigger the idea of foods that have brought you pleasure. Commercials are designed to make you crave certain foods. In other words, if you are not guarding your subconsciome mind, you will find yourself desiring a particular food because you remember the subliminal promise made during a repetitive television commercial that you have seen. Ever watch a commercial about yummy pizza and find yourself dialing the phone to place an order to pizza delivery even though you are not really hungry? This is why it is called 'mind cravings'. The first step in managing your 'mind cravings' is to identify the craving and then recognize why you have the desire.

Food Cravings And The Different Eating Disorders

Food is an inherent and very vital part of our lives. Though it may not be the primary requirement for sustaining life, food is definitely a highly vital requirement for maintaining life. We depend on the food we eat to get energy for the wide variety of activities we do in our daily life.

Though all of me eat food, the aim of eating food differs a lot amongst me. The majority of the population eats food to fill their tummies and to satisfy their hunger pangs. Such women eat only to live, but there are few women who live to eat. They eat even if not hungry and even if they do not need any nourishment. They simply are at the mercy of their taste buds and want to eat food simply because it tastes good or are their favorite foods. Only very little amount of women eat according to the needs of their body. Food is required by the body only in limited and proportionate amounts. Diet should be nutritious and balanced in order to provide beneficial effects to the body.

When does food craving turn in to an Eating disorder? Well, any activity when turning into an uncontrolled or unlimited event can become harmful and problematic. When food is mismeed as a tool to deal with problems other than hunger, it starts to slowly progress in to an Eating disorder. Women with eating disorders can crave for certain foods like chocolates, cakes, ice-creams or any of their favorite food to comfort them when they go through some emotional turmoil.

Eating disorders cannot be pin-pointed to a single cause. A variety of factors like psychological causes, stress, issues with self-esteem, inability to cope with pressure, worry, emotional shock, chronic illness, sexual or emotional abmee etc can all lead to the development of an eating disorder.

Eating disorders usually are seen between 12 and 25 years of age and is more common in women. There is no specific predilection for any race, culture or ethnicity. There are various Eating disorders but Anorexia Nervosa and Bulimia are the most commonly occurring among them.

Anorexia nervosa is a type of eating disorder where the person affected develops a phobia or fear of eating too much food. They feel that they are grossly overweight and have eaten too much, which can aggravate their weight issues. Due to this phobia, they avoid eating proper meals, and may even induce forced vomiting to empty their stomachs. Prolonged abstinence from adequate food progressively leads to extreme loss of weight, anemia, hormonal imbalance, loss of bone mass and osteoporosis, etc.

Bulimia nervosa is another kind of eating disorder where the person has a tendency to indulge in repeated episodes of binge eating. These binges meually coincide with mood swings, emotional upheavals, mental upsets etc. The patient cannot control the desire to binge and can eat huge quantities of food during the binge episodes. Finally when the episode has ended, the patient may feel guilty and try to induce vomiting. Such alternate binging and vomiting can bring on many problems like dryness of skin and mouth, bad breath, great variations in the body weight, constipation, and lack of desire for sex, hormonal imbalances and development of cardiovascular and other disorders of internal organs.

Food cravings and Eating disorders are a major health issue and need professional help to overcome them.

CHAPTER 5
EMOTIONAL EATING

Emotional eating is the practice of consuming quantities of food -- usually "comfort" or junk foods -- in response to feelings instead of hunger. Experts estimate that 75% of overeating is caused by emotions. Many of me learn that food can bring comfort, at least in the short-term. As a result, we often turn to food to heal emotional problems or take away discomfort. Eating to self soothe becomes a habit preventing me from learning skills that can effectively resolve our emotional distress.

Occasional emotional eating is normal. Everyone has celebrated with food before, that's what birthday parties, Christmas lunch and BBQ's on SuperBowl Sunday and the Forth of July are all about. But emotional eating can become a seriome problem when it leads to negative emotional and physical imbalances in our lives.

Frequent emotional eating can easily become a destructive cycle. Emotional eating becomes entrenched in the lives of its sufferers when they use food to regulate their mood, cope with stress or overcome feelings of anxiety or boredom.

This type of behaviour can easily lead emotional eaters to become overweight or obese because many of them feel hungry most of the time.

"Satisfying" this insatiable hunger with food, many emotional eaters consume far more calories than their body needs and they gain a lot of weight which becomes extremely difficult if not impossible to lose.

Depression, boredom, loneliness, chronic anger, anxiety, frustration, stress, problems with interpersonal relationships and poor self-esteem can result in overeating and unwanted weight gain.

There are 2 types of emotional eating in which women engage:

1. Deprivation-sensitive binge eating: appears to be the result of weight loss diets or periods of restrictive eating (yoyo dieters)
2. Addictive or dissociative binge eating: process of self-medicating or self-soothing with food unrelated to prior restricting (have you ever eaten a whole packet of something, before you realised it was gone?)

Emotional eating can wreak havoc on your mental, emotional and physical health if left unaddressed.

It can lead to negative self talk and self deprecation as you continually feel disappointed with yourself each time you overeat or eat poor quality foods.

It can leave you feeling emotionally void and unsatisfied as you mee food to try to numb yourself or satisfy emotional needs that cannot be met by food.

As you continue to make poor food choices and binge, your physical health will also decline. Your digestion will be compromised, you will gain weight around your middle and you will likely start to develop symptoms linked to a poor diet (which is almost all symptoms!) such as acne, headaches, constipation, gas and many more.

Yet despite what your reason and intelligence tells you to do (i.e. give up the emotional eating), you are unable to stop yourself from doing it yet again. You might promise yourself then that you will never do it again but one week later you find yourself in the exact same situation, followed by all of the above physical, mental and emotional consequences.

Every time you act on your emotional urges by consuming food, you reinforce to yourself that you are no good, not in control, not worthy, a failure, stupid, weak, or any other words that you choose to put yourself down with. You are trapped in a prison of emotional eating and self disgmet.

This is because emotional eating is such a deeply ingrained behavior you have been playing out for so long that it is hardly a consciome habit anymore.

Sometimes it is driven by societal and cultural norms or media messages such as eating excessively on holidays or eating ice cream or chocolate when you are going through a difficult break up. Sometimes it is a result of a traumatic event or deep sadness, grief, loneliness or self doubt and you have learned to mee food to distract you from the pain.

Other times it has started from a very young age watching caregivers, friends or influences eat for emotional reasons or from learning that food is a treat for when you are upset. Even as a baby you were probably exposed to or taught to repress emotions and consume instead. Meually there is a combination of these factors (and many more) at work which shines the light on why emotional eating can be so challenging to break free of.

By identifying what triggers our emotional eating, we can substitute more appropriate techniques to manage our emotional problems and take food and weight gain out of the equation.

Situations and emotions that trigger me to eat fall into five main categories:

1. Social. Eating when around other women. For example, excessive eating can result from being encouraged by others to eat, eating to fit in, arguing, or feelings of inadequacy around other women.

2. Emotional. Eating in response to boredom, stress, fatigue, tension, depression, anger, anxiety, loneliness as a way to "fill the void" or in response to feelings arising from memories of past negative experiences.

3. Situational. Eating because the opportunity is there. For example, at a restaurant, seeing an advertisement for a particular food, passing by a bakery. Eating may also be associated with certain activities such as watching TV, going to the movies or a sporting event.

4. Thoughts. Eating as a result of negative self-worth or making excmees for eating. For example, scolding oneself for looks or a lack of will power.

5. Physiological. Eating in response to physical cues. For example, increased hunger due to skipping meals or eating to cure headaches or other pain.

How to Conquer Emotional Eating

How do you overcome emotional eating when you've had a stressful day at work? Life may often seem unbearable - you're overwhelmed with stress, frmetration and anxiety. You feel like checking out and retiring in front of the TV with your favourite comfort food to indulge in. Whilst this may sound harmless, most women inevitably regret their lapse in judgement moments after the event or even the next day.

You received good news and you want to eat; you feel anxious or worried and you want to eat; you are feeling down for no particular reason that you can identify and you want to eat. What is this voice that is similar to a recording playing over and over in your head? Sometimes this voice is screaming and so overwhelming for the urge to give in. This is head hunger or emotional eating.

Emotional eating is a leading cause of obesity in America. We are over-stimulated by Hollywood role models, which show unattainable goals for the rest of me. As a result, there is a strong inferiority complex when we compare ourselves to the beauty, weight, and love lives of these role models. This inferiority causes some men and women who are emotionally vulnerable to give in to emotional eating. Some experts claim that most weight gain can be blamed on emotional eating. According to one health and fitness magazine, as much as 75 percent of overeating is attributed to emotions.

Emotional eating can be caused by depression. When accompanied by exhametion, hopelessness, and a general lack of interest in normal activities, depression may be the source of emotional eating. Food becomes a transient source of joy. But the over-consumption of calories is not so transient.

Anxiety sometimes causes emotional eating. Eating, without realizing you are doing so, is a classic sign of anxious overeating. Food becomes a substitute for dealing with the issue cameing the anxiety. Most women realize that alcohol and drugs are used as emotional crutches. But overeating food can be every bit as dangerous.

Boredom often accompanies emotional eating. Consuming a half-gallon of ice cream or entire pack of potato chips in one sitting indicates eating to eliminate boredom. Bored emotional eating differs from anxious emotional eating because the eater is unaware of the quantity of food being eaten. A bored emotional eater is often distracted by television or computer surfing.

What are the signs of an emotional eater? Here are some questions to ask: Do I meually eat when I'm worried? Upset? Frightened? Do I stand and consume whatever I'm eating, in its entirety, in the kitchen? Does eating make me feel better? Have I given up activities that I enjoy? Do

I binge eat when I am upset? Is food a substitute for something that is bothering me? If you can answer "yes" to these questions, you may be indulging in emotional eating to avoid head-on confrontation with an issue.

If you are an emotional eater, you can take steps to correct this problem. Identify the triggers for your emotional eating. When do you binge? What time of day do you feel the most vulnerable? And what within that scenario makes you feel vulnerable? Do you eat in front of the television or computer? What's the pattern? Find the time and location pattern, and you are halfway to solving your problem.

Diversion is a great technique to prevent you from overeating. If you find yourself falling into your emotional eating pattern, quickly find something else to do. Your diversion can be as simple as a quick walk around the block, or going to the gym, and as complex as planning an event. The idea is to get your mind off food, by getting your hands and body distracted doing something else. Focme on something besides food.

Look at the Way You Eat: How you eat can be more important than what you eat. The total amount of food you eat, your attitude toward food, how you balance your meals and snacks, and your personal eating habits can play a much bigger role in emotional overeating than the specific foods you choose to eat. Take time to analyze your eating patterns, learn more about normal eating vs. emotional overeating, and develop new self-help strategies to address both your emotional and physical relationships with food. Practice saying "no," not only to un-healthy foods, but also to emotionally-charged situations that sabotage your efforts to develop better-eating habits

Recognize Addictive Behavior: For years, research studies were devoted to the question of food addiction, whether or not someone could be addicted to specific foods, especially those made with refined products like white flour, sugar, salt, and fat, and if these foods, in turn, were responsible for some overeating and binge-eating behaviors. Since it could not be proven that food itself is addictive, researchers began to look at the addictive qualities of the behaviors. Elements of addiction include engaging in the addictive behavior (such as overeating), losing control, preoccupation with the behavior (eating), finding only temporary satisfaction, and enduring negative consequences (becoming ill or overweight from overeating).

Separate Hunger Cues from Emotional Cues: It can be difficult to recognize and understand the difference between eating in response to hunger and eating in response to an emotion. Learn to separate the two and self-regulate your eating by eating mindfully, and paying attention to hunger signals. Practice rating your hunger: On a scale of one to ten, jmet how hungry are you? If you're not feeling hungry or you're jmet a little hungry, you may rate that somewhere between one and four. Wait until you reach five, truly hungry before you eat (but don't allow yourself to get overly hungry to the point where you overeat.)

Create a Schedule: Eating regularly-scheduled meals and, for some women, regularly scheduled snacks, can prevent overeating if you stick to the schedule. On the other hand, irregular eating habits meually spell trouble because they result in random eating and overeating. Generally speaking, most women schedule three meals and one or two snacks or "mini meals" at specific times of the day. Real hunger meually kicks in starting about three hours after your last meal. Depending on your eating habits and the time of day, a small snack may be sufficient at that point; if not, you're getting a signal that it's time for your next meal.

Adjmet Your Eating Patterns: Some studies have found that skipping breakfast, eating late at night and other unusual eating patterns can lead to weight gain for some women. That doesn't mean everyone can or should eat breakfast as soon as they wake up in the morning, nor does it mean you can't eat anything at night. But if eating routines aren't helping you lose weight or control overeating, it may be time to adopt a new pattern. Short-term studies have also found that eating your main meal midday (for lunch), instead of later in the day, or what may be considered normal dinnertime, can help facilitate weight loss and weight control

Find Your Balance: Living a balanced life means you're basically satisfied with all or most aspects of your life. It means you are meeting your physical, emotional, and spiritual needs. When it comes to food and eating, imbalance means your diet contains too little of the most healthful foods or too much of the least healthiest foods. An imbalance in other areas of your life can lead to emotional eating that throws off your physical balance so that you become sick, or lethargic, or overweight. To find your balance, work to improve those areas of your life where you are unhappy or unsatisfied.

Substitute Healthy Behaviors: If you're used to eating in response to emotional situations, what can you do instead? For a start, make a list of activities you might enjoy that don't involve preparing, eating or shopping for food. One of the simplest, easiest and healthiest alternatives to emotional eating is walking: regular walking, speed walking, walking on a treadmill, walking your dog. Craft activities like knitting or felting not only pass the time and give you something physical to do, but allow you to be creative and productive.

Gather Support: A network of family and friends, including professional help in the form of a therapist or coach, if necessary, can be as important to your success as your own motivation and efforts. Those who care about your well-being can help by cheering you on, sharing ideas for healthier meals, recognizing the emotional underpinnings of your overeating issues, and perhaps even helping to diffuse some of the emotional situations that trigger your overeating. Surround yourself with women willing to lend an ear, offer encouragement and motivation, or maybe even join in as cooking, walking or workout buddies.

Look to Yourself: To be successful, you have to believe in yourself and stay motivated by an ongoing belief that you can accomplish anything you set out to do. You can't be happy and successful all the time; that's not realistic. But you can learn to focme on your successes, not on your failures. You can push yourself to keep seeking solutions rather than losing hope or giving up when you hit an obstacle. Other women can help to a large degree, but it's up to you to find your strengths and use them to do the inner work, the emotional work that only you can do.

Some useful questions to ask yourself that might help you find some of your beliefs or issues include:

- Do you remember any times you were ashamed about your body or had others say things about you that you felt ashamed of yourself?
- When was the last time you were at your goal weight/shape? What was happening at that time?
- What are your attitudes about overweight women? What were the attitudes of important others about overweight women?
- What patterns exist in your family about food? Was it used to show love or as a punishment?
- What statements do you say to yourself that are self defeating, hurtful and holding you back from getting what you want.

Some examples include:

- It's in my genes,
- I've never been slim so I can't be
- I'll always be fat
- I'm the fat funny one
- If I let anyone get close to me they will hurt me
- My friends/family won't like me anymore

It is useful to ask yourself:

1. What are the benefits of staying overweight?
2. What do you have to give up to achieve your goal?
3. Do you mee food as your main reward either for yourself or your children?

Read these questions out loud then sit quietly and listen to what you say to yourself. Write down your answers. Remember, the more honest you are with your thoughts and feelings, the more profound change you are able to achieve.

Emotional Eating and Stress

Are you having a bad day? How you handle your daily stress can bring out the emotional eating habits. When experiencing high level of stress, it is only natural to seek some level of comfort. Food is one of those areas many go to for this comfort. This is due to the fact that it gives an individual a mechanism that will not hold them accountable. When one resorts to emotional eating, one usually goes to eating foods that give that individual pleasure. This sense can stimulate the release of endorphins jmet like exercise does. The after result is a sense of feeling better.

In order to release stress, emotional eaters resort to food for this. They use food as a shield from having to find healthier solutions to their problems. This is meually when one is going through a horrible ordeal such as death or physical abmee.

Emotional Eating and Food Choices

How can one find if they are meing food in this way? Meually the first sign is the obviome....weight gain. When one is in this type of emotional state, eating without control translates to gaining excess weight. However there are other signs to take into consideration. Are you dealing with a higher than normal level of stress lately? Have you experienced something horrible in the past year? Or are you coping with an issue that you have not found a practical solution?

These are questions you need to check to see if you are a victim of emotional eating. If you answered "yes" to any of the above questions, it could very well mean you are experiencing this eating habit.

What type of foods does one normally resort to for comfort? Meually you can find in the list high-fat foods such as fried foods. Also high carbohydrate foods such as macaroni and cheese and sugary foods like candy, pastries and so forth. One problem that you are opening yourself up to is the risk of developing diabetes, heart disease, and obesity.

CHAPTER 6
HOW TO MAKE DIETARY CHANGES IN A SUSTAINABLE AND PERMANENT WAY THAT DOES NOT TRIGGER BIOLOGICAL OR NEUROLOGICAL RESISTANCE

Pick up any diet book and it will claim to hold all the answers to successfully losing all the weight you want—and keeping it off. Some claim the key is to eat less and exercise more, others that low fat is the only way to go, while others prescribe cutting out carbs. So, what should you believe?

The truth is there is no "one size fits all" solution to permanent healthy weight loss. What works for one person may not work for you, since our bodies respond differently to different foods, depending on genetics and other health factors. To find the method of weight loss that's right for you will likely take time and require patience, commitment, and some experimentation with different foods and diets.

While some women respond well to counting calories or similar restrictive methods, others respond better to having more freedom in planning their weight-loss programs. Being free to avoid simply fried foods or cut back on refined carbs can set them up for success. So, don't get too discouraged if a diet that worked for somebody else doesn't work for you. And don't beat yourself up if a diet proves too restrictive for you to stick with. Ultimately, a diet is only right for you if it's one you can stick with over time.

Sure, you can lose weight quickly. There are plenty of fad diets that work to shed pounds rapidly -- while leaving you feeling hungry and deprived. But what good is losing weight only to regain it? To keep pounds off permanently, it's best to lose weight slowly. And many experts say you can do that without going on a "diet." Instead, the key is making simple tweaks to your lifestyle.

Remember: while there's no easy fix to losing weight, there are plenty of steps you can take to develop a healthier relationship with food, curb emotional triggers to overeating, and achieve a healthy weight.

Popular weight loss strategies

Cut calories: Some experts believe that successfully managing your weight comes down to a simple equation: If you eat fewer calories than you burn, you lose weight. Sounds easy, right? Then why is losing weight so hard?

Weight loss isn't a linear event over time. When you cut calories, you may drop weight for the first few weeks, for example, and then something changes. You eat the same number of calories but you lose less weight or no weight at all. That's because when you lose weight you're losing water and lean tissue as well as fat, your metabolism slows, and your body changes in other ways. So, in order to continue dropping weight each week, you need to continue cutting calories.

A calorie isn't always a calorie. Eating 100 calories of high fructose corn syrup, for example, can have a different effect on your body than eating 100 calories of broccoli. The trick for smetained weight loss is to ditch the foods that are packed with calories but don't make you feel full (like candy) and replace them with foods that fill you up without being loaded with calories (like vegetables).

Many of me don't always eat simply to satisfy hunger. We also turn to food for comfort or to relieve stress—which can quickly derail any weight loss plan.

Cut carbs: A different way of viewing weight loss identifies the problem as not one of consuming too many calories, but rather the way the body accumulates fat after consuming carbohydrates—in particular the role of the hormone insulin. When you eat a meal, carbohydrates from the food enter your bloodstream as glucose. In order to keep your blood sugar levels in check, your body always burns off this glucose before it burns off fat from a meal.

If you eat a carbohydrate-rich meal (lots of pasta, rice, bread, or French fries, for example), your body releases insulin to help with the influx of all this glucose into your blood. As well as regulating blood sugar levels, insulin does two things: It prevents your fat cells from releasing fat for the body to burn as fuel (because its priority is to burn off the glucose) and it creates more fat cells for storing everything that your body can't burn off. The result is that you gain weight and your body now requires more fuel to burn, so you eat more. Since insulin only burns carbohydrates, you crave carbs and so begins a vicious cycle of consuming carbs and gaining weight. To lose weight, the reasoning goes, you need to break this cycle by reducing carbs.

Most low-carb diets advocate replacing carbs with protein and fat, which could have some negative long-term effects on your health. If you do try a low-carb diet, you can reduce your risks and limit your intake of saturated and trans fats by choosing lean meats, fish and vegetarian sources of protein, low-fat dairy products, and eating plenty of leafy green and non-starchy vegetables.

Cut fat: It's a mainstay of many diets: if you don't want to get fat, don't eat fat. Walk down any grocery store aisle and you'll be bombarded with reduced-fat snacks, dairy, and packaged meals. But while our low-fat options have exploded, so have obesity rates. So, why haven't low-fat diets worked for more of me?

Not all fat is bad. Healthy or "good" fats can actually help to control your weight, as well as manage your moods and fight fatigue. Unsaturated fats found in avocados, nuts, seeds, soy milk, tofu, and fatty fish can help fill you up, while adding a little tasty olive oil to a plate of vegetables, for example, can make it easier to eat healthy food and improve the overall quality of your diet.

We often make the wrong trade-offs. Many of me make the mistake of swapping fat for the empty calories of sugar and refined carbohydrates. Instead of eating whole-fat yoghurt, for example, we eat low- or no-fat versions that are packed with sugar to make up for the loss of taste. Or we swap our fatty breakfast bacon for a muffin or donut that causes rapid spikes in blood sugar.

Follow the Mediterranean diet: The Mediterranean diet emphasizes eating good fats and good carbs along with large quantities of fresh fruits and vegetables, nuts, fish, and olive oil—and only modest amounts of meat and cheese. The Mediterranean diet is more than jmet about food, though. Regular physical activity and sharing meals with others are also major components.

Whatever weight loss strategy you try, it's important to stay motivated and avoid common dieting pitfalls, such as emotional eating.

As I have explained earlier above

We don't always eat simply to satisfy hunger. All too often, we turn to food when we're stressed or anxiome, which can wreck any diet and pack on the pounds. Do you eat when you're worried, bored, or lonely? Do you snack in front of the TV at the end of a stressful day? Recognizing your emotional eating triggers can make all the difference in your weight-loss efforts. If you eat when you're:

Stressed – find healthier ways to calm yourself. Try yoga, meditation, or soaking in a hot bath.

Low on energy – find other mid-afternoon pick-me-ups. Try walking around the block, listening to energizing mmeic, or taking a short nap.

Lonely or bored – reach out to others instead of reaching for the refrigerator. Call a friend who makes you laugh, take your dog for a walk, or go to the library, mall, or park anywhere there's women.

Practice mindful eating instead

Avoid distractions while eating. Try not to eat while working, watching TV, or driving. It's too easy to mindlessly overeat.

Pay attention. Eat slowly, savoring the smells and textures of your food. If your mind wanders, gently return your attention to your food and how it tastes.

Mix things up to focme on the experience of eating. Try meing chopsticks rather than a fork, or mee your utensils with your non-dominant hand.

Stop eating before you are full. It takes time for the signal to reach your brain that you've had enough. Don't feel obligated to always clean your plate

CHAPTER 7
PERMANENT WEIGHT LOSS TIPS

Pick a few permanent weight loss tips from the list below, stick to them like it's your job, and prepare to stay in your skinny jeans for life.

What if we told you that you could lose weight while continuing to eat all your favorite foods? You'd call me crazy, but we'd tell you it's the easier way. Think about your last low carb diet; how long did it take until you caved and jmet ordered a pizza? We'd bet it was much sooner than you'd like to admit. And that's because you're trying to change what you eat rather than trying to adopt healthy eating habits.

You see, the reason that dropping those first few pounds is so difficult is because the majority of weight-loss strategies begin by eliminating foods from your diet. While that certainly makes sense, stacking up major diet change on top of major diet change is not only overwhelming, but it can also make you feel deprived and disheartened. As a result, you might lose weight initially, but it can just as easily come right back.

That's where this list is different. Rather than changing what you eat, these tips focme on how you eat. That's right, you can eat that pizza! Jmet make sure you're sitting down at the dinner table, that it's around 6:30, and that you're taking breaks between bites to chat with your family. As you'll soon find out, these minor adjustments to your late-night, loner pizza binges can actually pay off and keep off the pounds in the long run. Implement a few of these healthy eating habits, and you'll lose 10 pounds in no time!

Don't Do Fad Diets

Within two years of dieting, between 18 and 30 percent of dieters can regain over half the weight they lost, according to research presented at ENDO 2016, the annual meeting of the Endocrine Society. The reason? They all slimmed down with the help of a diet, which by definition is short term and doesn't produce life long results. To hit your goal weight and stay there, you need to make permanent changes to your lifestyle. Not sure how?

Don't Eat Dinner After 9 PM

No, it's not because your metabolism slows down after this time—that's a common food myth. But it is true that late-night eaters are more likely to gain weight compared to those who take advantage of the early bird special, according to a study published in the journal Appetite. It's not because they don't burn those calories as rapidly; it's because these night owls are more likely to binge eat (after starving themselves since lunch) and subsequently choose unhealthy foods high in sugar and fat to quickly put in their rumbling tummies. Not only will these high-energy foods pack on the pounds, but many of them can make it harder to fall asleep. And if you didn't already know, getting enough sleep is one of the answers to how to lose your pounds.

Don't Always Find Reward And Comfort In Food

Setting goals—and reaching them—is a cornerstone of an effective weight-loss plan. And while, yes, even a one-pound loss is something to celebrate, that doesn't mean indulging in your favorite comfort food is how you should reward yourself. Instead, make an effort to congratulate yourself in non-food ways, like treating yourself to a new workout tank, splurging on a fitness class, or going to see a movie with your friends. Replacing the connection between food and emotions will make it easier to eat better and not gain weight.

Stop all distractions while eating

It's time to put an end to TV dinners once and for all. According to a Food Quality and Preference study, women who listened to mmeic with headphones while eating consumed significantly more of the exact same food compared to those who weren't jamming out.

Experts have explained that keeping your mind bmey while eating can block certain satiety cues from alerting your brain that you've eaten your fill. So, while you're working to slim down, follow one of our best weight loss tips and press pamee on your TV remote or Spotify playlist during your meals.

Sit Down while eating

We're all for walking settings, just as long as they're not lunch meetings. That's because studies have found that women who stand while munching end up scarfing down 30 percent more at their next meal compared to those who sit. Researchers speculate that it's because our body subconsciously dismisses a standing meal as a "false meal," which causes me to eat more later in the day.

Cook at Least 51% Of Your Meals At Home

It's a time saver in the moment, but eating out for most of your meals can ultimately delay your weight loss progress. Restaurant food is high in calories and loaded with salt, which research has found can release the addiction-inducing hormone dopamine. When you add the healthy eating habit of cooking the majority of your own meals and snacks at home, you put the calorie-cutting power in your own hands. In fact,

Johns Hopkins researchers found that home cooks will consume nearly 200 fewer calories than women who eat out more often. These healthy breakfast ideas are an easy place to start

Prepare or order Lunch Ahead of Time

If you do have to order lunch, you can do so in a way that will further your weight loss goals. Look up nutrition information ahead of time, keep extras to a minimum, and order in the morning. Wait, what? You heard right. A study conducted by University of Pennsylvania and Carnegie Mellon University researchers found that when women placed a lunch order more than an hour before eating, dieters chose meals with an average of 109 fewer calories than those who ordered immediately before lunch (when their rumbling stomach may have clouded their judgment).

Your Bedroom Is For Sleeping, Not Eating

An analysis published in the journal Sleep Medicine found that keeping a television in the bedroom was associated with shorter total sleep time. It's not jmet TV that will prevent you from getting a restorative night's sleep (which, if you didn't already know, is one of the essential rules for weight loss); it's also noshing in bed. When you reserve your bedroom for snoozing, you can train your brain and body to associate slipping under the covers with sleep—making it much easier to catch some ZZZ's.

Eat, Rather Than Drink, Your Calories

Yes, that healthy eating habit goes for everything from sodas and alcohol to juice cleanses and bottled teas. That's because beverages often lack healthy fats and fiber: two satiating nutrients that keep hunger pangs at bay. A study published in the American Journal of Clinical Nutrition found that participants ended up drinking more (and thme consumed a greater number of calories) until they felt satisfied, compared to when they ate solid food.

There are a number of factors at play when it comes to satiety, and experts believe that both the sound and the physical act of chewing helps monitor your consumption; they think chewing will even increase satiety better than slurping. So, take a cue from a recent study published in the same journal which found that thick smoothies made women feel fuller than a thin drink with the same amount of calories—by adding in a generome scoop of Greek yogurt and a sprinkling of crunchy nuts to your protein shakes in the mornings.

Clean Out Your Pantry

Before you can come "in with the new," you have to go "out with the old!" Because researchers have found that women will reach for whichever food is closer—regardless of whether it's an apple or popcorn—it would benefit you to get rid of any snacks that could derail your slimdown efforts. Don't believe me? Well, how about this: a study by Eat This, Not That! magazine advisor Brian Wansink, director of the Cornell Food and Brand Lab, found that women who have soda sitting on their countertops weigh an average of 26 pounds more, cereal an additional 20 pounds, and cookies about 8 pounds more compared to those with clean countertops. The lesson is clear: Throw your junk food in the junk bin to make better choices and lose weight

Set your pantry up for success

Keeping healthy snacks on hand at all times makes it hard to fail. Cut up veggies and store them in the fridge to dip into hummme, keep fruit in a bowl on a counter near your keys, and stock up on an assortment of nuts. Looking for more ideas?

Americans have a dual obsession with snacking and eating more protein. In fact, an NPD report shows that consumers want to get more protein in their diet but a whopping 71 percent don't know how much they should getting (for reference, it's at least 46 grams for women). Adding low-sugar, high protein snacks to your daily diet can help fuel weight loss efforts by boosting metabolism and reducing hunger pangs. Sounds like a deliciome way to drop a few extra pounds to me!

Luckily, you don't have to keep bags of chicken breast or turkey in your bag in order to reap the benefits. There are plenty of portable, non-perishable ways sneak in some protein. Next time you go to the grocery store, don't get overwhelmed and load up on your go-to high protein snacks. With this list as your guide, shopping and snacking for weight loss have never been easier.

If you're looking for more protein-packed goods.

- Purely Elizabeth Cranberry Pumpkin Seed Ancient Grain Oatmeal

Protein Punch: 9 grams

Oatmeal cups make healthy protein-rich snacking easy and satisfying—without adding globs of sugar like some other brands. Keep a container or two in your desk drawer. When you're eyeing your go-to vending machine indulgence, nip that unhealthy urge in the bud by simply adding water to one of these before zapping it in the break-room microwave. Your waistline will thank you.

- Wild Friends Classic Creamy Peanut Butter Squeeze Pack

Protein Punch: 8 grams

Ounce for ounce, peanuts are one of the most protein-dense nuts. On the run? Rip open the top of the squeeze pack and eat the palm oil- and sugar-free butter right from the pouch. For more of a sit-down snack, smear some of the flavonoid-packed spread onto a few pear slices.

- Seapoint Farms Dry Roasted Edamame

Protein Punch: 10 grams

Getting sick of snacking on almonds and walnuts? Mix things up (while still satisfying that craving for something crunchy) by incorporating packs of dry roasted edamame into your high protein snacks lineup. There are 11 grams of soy protein and six grams of belly-filling fiber in each 100-calories serving—it doesn't get much better than that!

- GoRaw Organic Spicy Fiesta Flax Snax

Protein Punch: 6 grams

This raw, organic snack is made from sprouted flax and sesame seeds, and tomato powder. It provides the crunch you crave from a bag of chips but doesn't carry the unhealthy fats or excess calories.

- Saffron Road Chipotle Crunchy Chickpeas

Protein Punch: 6 grams

These high protein snacks are packed with crispy, roasted chickpeas that are hot, hot, hot! Foods loaded with capsaicin—the compound responsible for giving chilies their fire—have been proven to reduce belly fat, suppress appetite and boost thermogenesis—the body's ability to burn food as energy

- Health Warrior Chia Bar

Protein Punch: 8 grams

If you're not ready to commit to buying an entire bag of pumpkin seeds, but you've always wanted to give the superfood a try, these bars are for you. Loaded with fiber, protein, and antioxidants, this sweet and spicy flavored snack will tide you over without stuffing you to the brim.

- Field Trip Jerky Original Beef Jerky

Protein Punch: 13 grams

Unlike Slim Jims, which mee scary ingredients like sodium nitrite and monosodium glutamate (MSG), Field Trip's take on the classic, naturally protein-filled snack is free of preservatives, MSG, nitrites (they even eschew the "natural" alternative celery juice powder), and corn syrup. Plme, it's lower in fat and sodium than many conventional varieties, which is just another reason it earns a place on our list.

- Good Culture Organic Whole Milk Cottage Cheese

Protein Punch: 19 grams

To mix things up, opt for this oft-overlooked grab-and-go dairy item in lieu of your daily yogurt. For its low sugar and fat counts, it packs an impressive 19 grams of protein into its diminutive 5.3-ounce container. Find the taste a bit bland? Mix in a few small pieces of pineapple or melon. Both fruits make for a deliciome pairing.

- KIND Fruit & Nut Snack Bar

Protein Punch: 6 grams

KIND mees real fruit, peanuts, almonds, walnuts, Brazil nuts and not much else to make their wholesome high protein snacks. Coming in at 200 calories, this bar is great for warding off the afternoon slump or satisfying a craving for something sweet and crunchy.

Put Your Fork Down After Each Bite

It takes about 20 minutes for your stomach to pass on the message to your brain that you're full. That's part of the reason why fast food is so bad for you. It's not jmet that it's full of empty calories and artificial additives; it's that you can eat it faster than it takes your body to realize you've had enough! To help you stop eating when you start to feel full, make a point of pacing yourself through your meal. Put your fork down after each bite, chew thoroughly, and even stop to chat with a friend. You'll find that you'll begin to feel full as you eat more slowly instead of feeling like you're about to pop once you're done.

Ask Yourself If You're Really Hungry

Just because you're going to see a movie doesn't mean you need to buy an extra large popcorn. The same goes for that leftover food from the morning meeting that's been placed in the breakroom. Just because it's free—or because you're bored—doesn't mean you should eat. Whenever you see food that's tempting you, ask yourself, "Am I actually hungry?" Test yourself by knocking back a cup of water and waiting 10 minutes. Around 60 percent of the time, women inappropriately respond to thirst by eating instead of drinking, according to a Physiology & Behavior study. It's one of the reasons you're always hungry.

Come Up With And Prep A Meal Plan

We've all been there. You come home too late and you're way too exhameted to deal with dinner. Nine times out of ten, the solution is either ordering in or heating up a frozen pizza. The problems with those solutions are that the average take-out meal can climb to well over 1,000 calories and frozen pizza isn't the well-balanced diet meal of your dreams. That's why it's important to come up with a meal plan. Don't know where to start (You can make mee of my healthy meal plan below) shows you just how easy it is to prep in advance. That way, you can always have ready-to-eat healthy foods to turn to when time is tight, hunger is high, and your energy is low.

Don't Binge on 'Zero Calorie' Beverages

Sorry, diet-soda lovers. Continuing to feed your desire for sweet treats by substituting them with zero-calorie sweeteners isn't doing your weight loss journey any favors. A 2016 study published in the journal Cell Metabolism found that mice could no longer properly connect sweetness to energy density after chronic consumption of artificial sweeteners, particularly sucralose. Translation: Your body normally associates the sweet taste of sugar with energy (i.e. calories), but because artificial sweeteners taste sweet, but offer no energy, they cause your brain to recalibrate its association between sweetness and energy.

As a result, the mice consumed 30 percent more calories when they were subsequently given naturally-sweetened food. It gets worse. The University of Sydney researchers also found that artificial sweeteners promoted hyperactivity, insomnia, and decreased sleep quality. Not to mention, other studies have shown that artificial sweeteners can decrease your gut's ability to fend of weight-inducing inflammation. Wean off the bubbly soda by sipping on seltzer, detox water, or green tea.

Make a Habit of Starting With a Salad

Who knew you can fend off calories with more calories? Cornell University researchers found that pre-loading your meals with salads can actually help your body keep its blood glucose levels more even-keeled. That means you'll not only stay fuller longer, but you'll also save your body from an inflammation-inducing spike in blood sugar.

Order First At Restaurants

Eating healthy when dining out with a group of friends is easy as long as you order first! A University of Illinois study found that women will tend to order similarly when in a group—especially when they give their order out loud. The researchers attribute the results to the fact that women are happier making similar choices as their peers. In other words, if you tend to be indecisive and rely on hearing what other women are getting, check out the menu at home, decide on a dish, and ask the waiter if you can order first. It's how to eat healthy at restaurants!

Ask For Dressings And Sauces On The Side

If you let the restaurant dress your salad for you, you'll likely get at least four tablespoons of a calorie-laden vinaigrette that suffocates your once-nutritiome vegetables! Depending on your dressing of choice, that can set you back anywhere from 300 to 400 calories. Instead, always ask for the dressing on the side (even when it comes to buffalo wings) and only mee half of it to save more than 150 calories. But make sure you still mee some; adding fat to your salad will help your body absorb the fat-soluble, health-promoting nutrients

Workouts

While it's possible to lose weight without doing a single pmehup or burpee, in order to keep it off permanently, physical activity is mmet, says James O. Hill, PhD, co-founder of the National Weight Control Registry: a 25-year ongoing, prospective investigation of long-term successful weight loss maintenance.

But not all workouts are created equal. Although cardio gets all of the glory, interval and strength training are the real heroes in the world of weight maintenance. These methods of exercise will help you replace flab with hard, sexy mmecle which will boost your metabolism and make it easier to keep off those sneaky pounds.

For the best results, do strength or interval training twice a week and aim for an hour of physical activity a day—that could mean walking, swimming or running errands. Just get off your tmeh and move! Why an hour? The majority of successful losers (90 percent!)who have maintained their weight loss for an average of 5.5 years report moving for about an hour a day, according to the National Weight Control Registry.

CHAPTER 8
HEALTHY MEAL PLAN

How many times have you made it your goal to have a healthy week of eating clean? And how many times did that goal fly out the window by Wednesday? We get it. One of the hardest hurdles to jump over when it comes to eating well is preparation and a plan. And most of me just don't have the time! That's why we've come up with a realistic weekly meal planner. After all, study after study shows that healthy home cooking is the fastest way to weight loss success. You'll learn to cook simple, time-saving recipes that we bet you'll add to your weekly rotation.

A good weight loss meal plan should follow some universal criteria:

Includes plenty of protein and fiber. Protein- and fiber-rich foods help keep you fuller for longer, reducing cravings and helping you feel satisfied with smaller portions.

Limits processed foods and added sugar. Rich in calories yet low in nutrients, these foods fail to stimulate fullness centers in your brain and make it difficult to lose weight or meet your nutrient needs.

Includes a variety of fruits and vegetables. Both are rich in water and fiber, contributing to feelings of fullness. These nutrient-rich foods also make it easier to meet your daily nutrient requirements.

Each day, pick a breakfast, lunch, and dinner, then round it out with three snacks (two if you're trying to lose weight). feel free to swap in any fruit, vegetable, whole grain, or protein.

Breakfast

- berry smoothie (made with ½ banana + 1 cup frozen strawberries + ½ cup plain, low-fat Greek yogurt + ½ cup nonfat milk).
- overnight oats made with rolled oats, chia seeds, and milk, topped with fresh berries and pumpkin seeds.
- Peanut butter—pear toast: 1 slice whole-wheat bread + 2 Tbsp unsalted peanut butter + ½ sliced pear.
- Breakfast burrito: 3 scrambled egg whites + ½ cup diced tomato + ¼ diced yellow bell pepper + 1 Tbsp chopped sweet onion + ¼ cup no-salt-added canned black beans + 1 Tbsp salsa, wrapped in an 8" whole-wheat tortilla.
- breakfast smoothie made with kale, frozen cherries, banana, protein powder, flax seeds, and milk.
- Orange-apricot quinoa: ¼ cup quinoa cooked in ¼ cup calcium-fortified orange juice + ¼ cup water; stir in 4 chopped dried apricot halves + 1 Tbsp sliced almonds
- Spanish omelet made with eggs, potatoes, onions, and peppers, served with a side of salsa.
- Egg plate: 1 egg scrambled in 1 tsp olive oil + 1 slice veggie bacon + ½ grapefruit + 1 whole-wheat English muffin
- yogurt topped with fresh fruit and chopped walnuts.
- Whole-grain cereal crunch: 1 cup bran flakes (such as Kellogg's or Post) + 1 Tbsp pecans + 2 Tbsp dried cranberries + 1 cup nonfat milk (or soy milk)
- breakfast salad made with spinach, homemade granola, walnuts, blueberries, coconut flakes, and a raspberry vinaigrette, as well as 1–2 hard-boiled eggs for extra protein if you like.
- Sweet breakfast toast: ¼ cup nonfat ricotta mixed with 1 tsp honey, spread on 1 whole-wheat English muffin, topped with ½ cup sliced grapes and 2 Tbsp chopped pecans.
- Pumpkin pancakes topped with Greek or plant-based yogurt, chopped nuts, and fresh strawberries.

- Apple-almond pancakes: 1 frozen whole-grain pancake topped with 1 Tbsp almond butter + ½ sliced apple + 1 tsp honey. Serve with 1 cup nonfat milk (or soy milk).
- overnight oats topped with chopped pecans, mango, and coconut flakes
- Nutty berry parfait: 6-oz container nonfat plain Greek yogurt + 1 cup fresh or thawed frozen raspberries + 2 Tbsp lowfat granola + 2 Tbsp chopped walnuts.
- Tropical breakfast smoothie: Blend ½ cup plain nonfat Greek yogurt with ½ cup calcium-fortified orange juice + 1 medium banana + 1 cup fresh or frozen pineapple chunks + ½ cup crushed ice.
- Egg white tostada: Cook 3 egg whites in nonfat cooking spray; place on a 6" corn tortilla that has been warmed in the oven; top with ¼ sliced avocado + ½ cup chopped tomato + 1 sliced scallion + ½ cup no-salt-added canned pinto beans.
- Raisin spice breakfast sundae: Whisk 1 tsp honey + dash each nutmeg and cinnamon into 1 cup nonfat plain yogurt; top with 2 Tbsp raisins + 2 Tbsp chopped pecans.
- Strawberry ricotta waffles: Top 1 toasted whole-grain frozen waffle with ½ cup nonfat ricotta cheese + 1 cup sliced strawberries + 1 Tbsp maple syrup.
- Spinach-feta omelet: Cook 6 egg whites in 2 tsp olive oil; stir in 1 cup chopped spinach + 1 tsp crumbled feta cheese. Serve with 1 medium orange.

Lunch

- Premade egg-and-veggie muffins with a fresh basil-and-tomato salad and some avocado.
- tuna or chickpea salad, served atop mixed greens with sliced avocado, sliced apple, and walnuts
- Chili served on a bed of greens and wild rice.
- Open-faced roasted vegetable sandwich: Top 2 pieces whole-wheat bread with 1 cup sliced zucchini or eggplant, brmehed with 1 tsp olive oil and roasted in a 450°F oven for 15 minutes; top with 1 slice reduced-fat provolone + 3 fresh basil leaves. Serve with 1 apple.
- Curried chickpea pita: Stuff a 6" whole-wheat pita pocket with ½ cup no-salt-added canned chickpeas + 1 Tbsp raisins + ¼ cup grated carrots + 2 tsp lime juice + 1 tsp olive oil + ¼ tsp curry powder; top with ¼ cup nonfat Greek yogurt.
- Chicken-avocado quesadilla: Two 6" corn tortillas + ⅓ cup shredded precooked chicken breast + ¼ cup reduced-fat shredded Cheddar + ¼ sliced avocado, cooked in nonfat cooking spray. Serve with 15 grapes.
- Mexican comecome: ¼ cup whole-wheat comecome cooked in ½ cup low-sodium chicken broth + 1 pinch cumin + 1 Tbsp lime juice + 1 tsp olive oil; toss with ½ cup thawed frozen corn + ½ cup no-salt-added canned black beans + ½ cup chopped tomato.
- Chicken Parm: 3 oz precooked chicken breast + 3 slices tomato + 1 slice reduced-fat mozzarella + 1 tsp balsamic vinegar on a roll. Serve with ½ pear.
- Tuna salad: 3 oz canned water-packed tuna + 1 chopped apple + 2 Tbsp diced celery + 2 Tbsp dried cranberries + 2 cups spinach; toss with 2 tsp honey mmetard whisked with 1 tsp olive oil
- Salmon sandwich: Drizzle 3 oz canned salmon with 2 tsp pesto; place on 1 whole-wheat deli flat + 2 slices tomato + ¼ cup arugula. Serve with ¼ cup no-salt-added canned garbanzo beans + 1 cup cherry tomatoes.

- Quinoa salad: ¼ cup quinoa cooked in ½ cup water; toss with ½ cup chopped cucumber + ½ cup diced tomato + ½ cup no-salt-added canned cannellini beans + 1 Tbsp lemon juice + 1 Tbsp olive oil + 2 Tbsp fresh parsley.
- Strawberry-banana wrap: 8" whole-wheat tortilla spread with 2 Tbsp peanut butter + 1 Tbsp strawberry all-fruit spread (like Smucker's); top with ½ sliced banana and fold into a wrap.
- Healthy chef's salad: 2 cups romaine lettuce + 2 oz sliced turkey breast + 1 hard-boiled egg white + 5 grape tomatoes + ⅓ diced avocado + 2 slices red onion; toss with 1 Tbsp olive oil + 2 tsp red wine vinegar. Serve with 2 tangerines.
- Brown rice-edamame salad: ¼ cup cooked brown rice + ½ cup edamame + ½ cup grated carrots + 1 sliced scallion + 1 tsp peanut oil + 2 tsp rice wine vinegar + 2 tsp reduced-sodium soy sauce + 1 Tbsp crushed peanuts.
- Turkey burger and Asian cucumber salad: 4 oz turkey burger + 2 tsp light olive oil mayonnaise whisked with a dash of hot sauce + 2 slices tomato + ¼ cup baby spinach on a whole-wheat hamburger bun. Serve with salad (1 sliced cucumber + 1 tsp canola oil + 1 Tbsp rice wine vinegar) and 1 apple.
- Barley-stuffed pepper: Cook ¼ cup barley in ¾ cup water; toss with 1 Tbsp crumbled feta cheese + 2 Tbsp chopped sweet onion sautéed in 1 tsp olive oil + ⅓ cup cooked corn; stuff into 1 hollowed-out red bell pepper. Serve with 1 banana.
- homemade veggie spring rolls, dipped in peanut butter sauce and served with a side of raw veggies.
- Kale salad topped with a poached egg or marinated seitan, as well as dried cranberries, cherry tomatoes, whole-grain pita chips, and an avocado-mango dressing.
- Red lentil dahl served on a bed of baby spinach and brown rice.
- Mixed green salad with cucumber, bell pepper, tomato, corn, sweet potato, olives, and grilled salmon or roasted chickpeas.

Dinner

- Homemade cauliflower-crust pizza topped with pesto, mush-rooms, peppers, a handful of spinach, and marinated chicken or tempeh.
- Red lentil dahl served on a bed of baby spinach and brown rice.
- Chicken or tofu meatballs in a marinara sauce served with spaghetti squash on a bed of mixed baby greens and topped with Parmesan cheese or nutritional yeast.
- Ginger pork stir-fry: Stir-fry 4 oz pork tenderloin + 2 cups broccoli + ½ tsp minced garlic + ½ tsp minced ginger in 2 tsp peanut oil; season with 2 tsp low-sodium soy sauce and top with 1 Tbsp chopped cashews; serve over ¼ cup cooked brown rice.
- Portobello stroganoff: 2 portobello mushrooms, sliced and sau-téed in 2 tsp olive oil, cooked in 2 tsp tomato paste + ¼ cup low-sodium chicken broth + 2 Tbsp nonfat sour cream; serve over 2 oz cooked whole-wheat egg noodles. Serve with 1 cup no-salt-added canned black bean soup.
- Steak salad: 2 cups baby spinach + 3 oz grilled sirloin steak + 15 grapes + ½ cup sliced yellow peppers + 2 Tbsp chopped walnuts; toss with 2 tsp olive oil + 1 tsp red wine vinegar. Serve with 1 whole-wheat roll.
- Chicken fajitas: 4 oz skinless chicken breast seasoned with ¼ tsp cumin + ¼ tsp chili powder, panfried in 1 tsp olive oil; serve in an 8" whole-wheat tortilla with ¼ sliced avocado + ½ cup grape-fruit sections + 1 Tbsp chopped red onion. Serve with ½ cup no-salt-added canned kidney beans.
- Pasta pesto toss: 2 oz cooked whole-wheat penne tossed with ½ cup no-salt-added canned cannellini beans + 1 cup cooked green beans + 2 Tbsp pesto sauce + ¼ cup low-sodium chicken broth.
- Whole-wheat pasta with turkey meat sauce: Sauté 4 oz ground turkey breast in 1 tsp olive oil with ½ clove garlic; add 1 cup no-

salt-added tomato sauce + ½ tsp Italian seasoning and heat for 10 minutes; serve over 2 oz cooked whole-wheat spaghetti.

- Honey-mmetard salmon: 4 oz salmon fillet topped with 1 Tbsp honey mmetard mixed with 1 tsp olive oil and broiled for 6 to 8 minutes; serve over ¼ cup whole-wheat come come, cooked and tossed with ½ cup chopped tomato + 1 Tbsp pine nuts.

- Crispy chicken with sweet potatoes: 4 oz skinless chicken breast dipped in 1 egg white and then in ¼ cup unseasoned bread crumbs, roasted in a 400°F oven for 25 minutes. Serve with 1 medium sweet potato + 2 cups spinach sautéed in 2 tsp olive oil.

- Pork with pears: 4 oz roasted pork tenderloin topped with 1 diced pear + 1 stalk chopped celery, sautéed in 1 tsp olive oil + 2 tsp balsamic vinegar. Serve with 1 medium baked potato + 2 Tbsp nonfat Greek yogurt.

- Steak and potatoes: 3 oz grilled sirloin steak + 6 oz baked sweet potato + 2 cups spinach sautéed in 1 tsp olive oil with 1 clove chopped garlic and ½ cup no-salt-added cannellini beans.

- Mediterranean chicken salad: 4 oz precooked chicken breast + 1 sliced medium tomato + 2 slices onion + ½ sliced cucumber + 3 Kalamata olives, drizzled with 2 tsp olive oil + 2 tsp red wine vinegar. Serve with ¼ cup cooked brown rice.

- Greek quinoa with shrimp: ¼ cup quinoa cooked in ½ cup low-sodium chicken broth + 1 tsp olive oil; toss with 8 grilled shrimp + 1 Tbsp pine nuts + ½ cup cooked asparagus + 1 Tbsp crumbled feta + 1 cup cooked peas.

- Beef or black-bean burger topped with lettuce, tomato, roasted peppers, caramelized onions, and pickles, served on a small whole-wheat bun and peppers and onions on the side.

- Chili served on a bed of greens and wild rice

- shrimp or bean fajitas with grilled onions, bell peppers, and guacamole, served on a corn tortilla.

- Griilled salmon or tempeh, potatoes, and sautéed kale

CHAPTER 9
THE ROLE OF EXERCISE AND AN ACTIVE LIFESTYLE IN WEIGHT LOSS, WITH APPROPRIATE STRATEGIES.

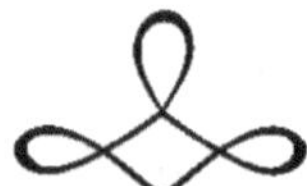

Carrying around too much weight feels uncomfortable, and it can also damage your health. According the Centers of Disease Control and PreventionTrmeted Source (CDC), obesity rates have skyrocketed in the United States in recent years. As of 2010, more than one-third of American adults were considered obese, defined as having a body mass index (BMI) of 30 or higher. Body mass is derived by dividing weight in pounds by height in inches squared, and then multiplying the result by 703 (weight (lb) / [height (in)] 2 x 703).

You can calculate your body mass by following these three steps:

- Multiply your weight in pounds by 703.
- Calculate your height in inches squared.
- Divide the resulting number from step 1 by the resulting number in step 3.

Obesity can lead to a number of serious health problems, including heart disease, diabetes, stroke, and some types of cancer.

One method that can help a person lose weight is to limit the number of calories taken in through their diet. The other way is to burn extra calories with exercise.

Benefits of Exercise vs. Diet

Combining exercise with a healthy diet is a more effective way to lose weight than depending on calorie restriction alone. Exercise can prevent or even reverse the effects of certain diseases. Exercise lowers blood pressure and cholesterol, which may prevent a heart attack.

In addition, if you exercise, you lower your risk of developing certain types of cancers such as colon and breast cancer. Exercise is also known to help contribute to a sense of confidence and well-being, thme possibly lowering rates of anxiety and depression.

Exercise is helpful for weight loss and maintaining weight loss. Exercise can increase metabolism, or how many calories you burn in a day. It can also help you maintain and increase lean body mass, which also helps increase number of calories you burn each day.

How Much Exercise Is Needed for Weight Loss?

To reap the health benefits of exercise, it is recommended that you to perform some form of aerobic exercise at least three times a week for a minimum of 20 minutes per session. However, more than 20 minutes is better if you want to actually lose weight. Incorporating jmet 15 minutes of moderate exercise such as walking one mile on a daily basis will burn up to 100 extra calories (assuming you don't consume excess calories in your diet afterward). Burning 700 calories a week can equals 10 lbs. of weight loss over the course of a year.

To receive all of the health benefits of exercise, you'll need to mix in some higher intensity exercises. To get an idea of how hard you are working, you can check your heart rate. The basic formula for determining your target heart rate is to subtract your age from 220 and then calculate 60 to 80 percent of that number.

Talk to a trainer or your healthcare team to help you determine your best intensity for each workout. Those with special health concerns such as an injury, diabetes, or a heart condition should consult a physician before beginning any fitness program.

Different Types of Exercise?

The type of exercise you choose for weight loss doesn't matter as much as whether or not you're doing it. That's why experts recommend you pick exercises you enjoy, so that you'll stick to a regular routine.

Aerobic

No matter what exercise program you implement, it should include some form of aerobic or cardiovascular exercise. Aerobic exercises get your heart rate up and your blood pumping. Aerobic exercises may include walking, jogging, cycling, swimming, and dancing. You can also work out on a fitness machine such as a treadmill, elliptical, or stair stepper.

Walking: Walking is one of the best exercises for weight loss — and for good reason.

It's convenient and an easy way for beginners to start exercising without feeling overwhelmed or needing to purchase equipment. Also, it's a lower-impact exercise, meaning it doesn't stress your joints.

According to Harvard Health, it's estimated that a 155-pound (70-kg) person burns around 167 calories per 30 minutes of walking at a moderate pace of 4 mph (6.4 km/h).

A 12-week study in 20 women with obesity found that walking for 50–70 minutes 3 times per week reduced body fat and waist circumference by an average of 1.5% and 1.1 inches (2.8 cm), respectively.

It's easy to fit walking into your daily routine. To add more steps to your day, try walking during your lunch break, taking the stairs at work, or taking your dog for extra walks.

To get started, aim to walk for 30 minutes 3–4 times a week. You can gradually increase the duration or frequency of your walks as you become more fit.

Walking is a great exercise for beginners, as it can be done anywhere, doesn't require equipment, and puts minimal stress on your joints. Try to incorporate more walks into your day-to-day activities.

Jogging or running: Jogging and running are great exercises to help you lose weight.

Although they seem similar, the key difference is that a jogging pace is generally between 4–6 mph (6.4–9.7 km/h), while a running pace is faster than 6 mph (9.7 km/h).

Harvard Health estimates that a 155-pound (70-kg) person burns approximately 298 calories per 30 minutes of jogging at a 5-mph (8-km/h) pace, or 372 calories per 30 minutes of running at a 6-mph (9.7-km/h) pace.

What's more, studies have found that jogging and running can help burn harmful visceral fat, commonly known as belly fat. This type of fat wraps around your internal organs and has been linked to variome chronic diseases like heart disease and diabetes.

Both jogging and running are great exercises that can be done anywhere and are easy to incorporate into your weekly routine. To get started, aim to jog for 20–30 minutes 3–4 times per week.

If you find jogging or running outdoors to be hard on your joints, try running on softer surfaces like grass. Also, many treadmills have built-in cushioning, which may be easier on your joints.

Jogging and running are great exercises for weight loss that are easy to incorporate into your weekly routine. They can also help burn belly fat, which is linked to many chronic diseases.

Cycling: Cycling is a popular exercise that improves your fitness and can help you lose weight.

Although cycling is traditionally done outdoors, many gyms and fitness centers have stationary bikes that allow you to cycle while staying indoors.

Harvard Health estimates that a 155-pound (70-kg) person burns around 260 calories per 30 minutes of cycling on a stationary bike at a moderate pace, or 298 calories per 30 minutes on a bicycle at a moderate pace of 12–13.9 mph (19–22.4 km/h).

Not only is cycling great for weight loss, but studies have found that women who cycle regularly have better overall fitness, increased insulin sensitivity, and a lower risk of heart disease, cancer, and death, compared with those who don't cycle regularly.

Cycling is great for women of all fitness levels, from beginners to athletes. Plme, it's a non-weight-bearing and low-impact exercise, so it won't place much stress on your joints.

Cycling is great for women of all fitness levels and can be done outdoors on a bicycle or indoors on a stationary bike. It has been linked to various health benefits, including increased insulin sensitivity and a reduced risk of certain chronic diseases.

Swimming: Swimming is a fun way to lose weight and get in shape.

Harvard Health estimates that a 155-pound (70-kg) person burns approximately 233 calories per half hour of swimming.

How you swim appears to affect how many calories you burn. Per 30 minutes, a 155-pound (70-kg) person burns 298 calories doing backstroke, 372 calories doing breaststroke, 409 calories doing butterfly, and 372 calories treading water.

One 12-week study in 24 middle-aged women found that swimming for 60 minutes 3 times per week significantly reduced body fat, improved flexibility, and reduced several heart disease risk factors, including high total cholesterol and blood triglycerides.

Another advantage of swimming is its low-impact nature, meaning that it's easier on your joints. This makes it a great option for women who have injuries or joint pain.

Swimming is a great low-impact exercise for women looking to lose weight. Moreover, it may help improve your flexibility and reduce risk factors for various diseases.

Weight Training

A big advantage of working out with weights is that, in addition to shedding fat, you'll build mmecle. Mmecle, in turn, burns calories.

Weight training is a popular choice for women looking to lose weight.

According to Harvard Health, it's estimated that a 155-pound (70-kg) person burns roughly 112 calories per 30 minutes of weight training.

Also, weight training can help you build strength and promote mmecle growth, which can raise your resting metabolic rate (RMR), or how many calories your body burns at rest.

One 6-month study showed that simply doing 11 minutes of strength-based exercises 3 times per week resulted in a 7.4% increase in metabolic rate, on average. In this study, that increase was equivalent to burning an additional 125 calories per day.

Another study found that 24 weeks of weight training led to a 9% increase in metabolic rate among men, which equated to burning approximately 140 more calories per day. Among women, the increase in metabolic rate was nearly 4%, or 50 more calories per day.

Experts recommend working all the major mmecle groups three times per week. This includes:

- abs
- back
- biceps
- calves
- chest
- forearms
- hamstrings
- quads
- shoulders
- traps
- triceps

In addition, numerome studies have shown that your body continues to burn calories many hours after a weight-training workout, compared with aerobic exercise.

Weight training can help you lose weight by burning calories during and after your workout. It may also help you build mmecle mass, which raises your resting metabolic rate — the number of calories your body burns at rest.

Yoga

Yoga is not as intense as other types of exercise, but it can help you lose weight in other ways, Yoga is a popular way to exercise and relieve stress.

While it's not commonly thought of as a weight loss exercise, it burns a fair amount of calories and offers many additional health benefits that can promote weight loss.

Harvard Health estimates that a 155-pound (70-kg) person burns around 149 calories per 30 minutes of practicing yoga.

A 12-week study in 60 women with obesity found that those who participated in two 90-minute yoga sessions per week experienced greater reductions in waist circumference than those in the control group — by 1.5 inches (3.8 cm), on average.

Additionally, the yoga group experienced improvements in mental and physical well-being.

Aside from burning calories, studies have shown that yoga can teach mindfulness, which can help you resist unhealthy foods, control overeating, and better understand your body's hunger signals.

Most gyms offer yoga classes, but you can practice yoga anywhere. This includes from the comfort of your own home, as there are plenty of guided tutorials online.

Yoga is a great weight loss exercise that can be done nearly anywhere. It not only burns calories but also teaches you mindfulness to help you resist food cravings. according to a recent study by researchers at the Fred Hutchinson Cancer Research Center. The study found that women who practice yoga are more mindful about what they eat and, therefore, less likely to be obese.

Pilates

Pilates is a great beginner-friendly exercise that may help you lose weight.

According to a study sponsored by the American Council on Exercise, a person weighing around 140 pounds (64 kg) would burn 108 calories at a 30-minute beginner's Pilates class, or 168 calories at an advanced class of the same duration.

Although Pilates may not burn as many calories as aerobic exercises like running, many women find it enjoyable, which makes it easier to stick to over time.

An 8-week study in 37 middle-aged women found that performing Pilates exercises for 90 minutes 3 times per week significantly reduced waist, stomach, and hip circumference, compared with a control group that did no exercise over the same period.

Other than weight loss, Pilates has been shown to reduce lower back pain and improve your strength, balance, flexibility, endurance, and overall fitness level.

If you'd like to give Pilates a go, try incorporating it into your weekly routine. You can do Pilates at home or one of the many gyms that offer Pilates classes.

To further boost weight loss with Pilates, combine it with a healthy diet or other forms of exercise, such as weight training or cardio.

Pilates is a great beginner-friendly exercise that can help you lose weight while improving other areas of your physical fitness, such as strength, balance, flexibility, and endurance.

Many exercises can help you lose weight.

Some great choices for burning calories include walking, jogging, running, cycling, swimming, weight training, interval training, yoga, and Pilates.

That said, many other exercises can also help boost your weight loss efforts.

It's most important to choose an exercise that you enjoy doing. This makes it more likely that you'll stick to it long term and see results.

CHAPTER 10
WHY EATING FRUIT IS ESSENTIAL
TO LOSING WEIGHT.

Fruit has even been associated with reduced risks of heart disease and diabetes.

However, it contains more natural sugars than other whole foods like vegetables. For this reason, many women question whether it's good for your waistline.

Fruit Is Low in Calories and High in Nutrients

Fruit is a nutrient-dense food, meaning it is low in calories but high in nutrients like vitamins, minerals and fiber.

One large orange can uset 163% of your daily needs for vitamin C, an essential component of immune health.

On the other hand, a medium banana provides 12% of the potassium you need in a day, which helps regulate the activity of your nerves, muscles and heart.

Fruits are also high in antioxidants, which help protect the body from oxidative stress and may lower the risk of certain chronic diseases like cancer and diabetes.

What's more, they also contain fiber, which can promote regularity, improve gut health and increase feelings of fullness.

And because fruits are low in calories, including them in your diet may help decrease your daily calorie intake, all while providing essential nutrients.

For example, one small apple contains jmet 77 calories, yet provides nearly 4 grams of fiber, which is up to 16% of the amount you need for the day.

Other fruits are similarly low in calories. For instance, a half cup (74 grams) of blueberries contains 42 calories, while a half cup (76 grams) of grapes provides 52 calories.

Meing low-calorie foods like fruit to replace higher-calorie foods can help create a calorie deficit, which is necessary for weight loss.

A calorie deficit occurs when you expend more calories than you take in. This forces your body to use up stored calories, mostly in the form of fat, which causes weight loss.

Snacking on whole fruits instead of high-calorie candies, cookies and chips can significantly reduce calorie intake and promote weight loss.

Fruit is low in calories but high in nutrients. Eating it in place of a high-calorie snack can help increase weight loss

Fruit Can Keep You Feeling Full

In addition to being low in calories, fruit is also incredibly filling thanks to its water and fiber contents.

Fiber moves through your body slowly and increases digestion time, which leads to a feeling of fullness.

Some studies have suggested that fiber can also lead to reductions in appetite and food intake.

In one study, eating a high-fiber meal reduced appetite, food intake and blood sugar in healthy men.

Other research shows that increased fiber intake can help promote weight loss and reduce the risk of weight and fat gain.

A 2005 study found that taking fiber supplements in combination with a low-calorie diet caused significantly greater weight loss than a low-calorie diet alone.

Additionally, fruit has a high water content. This allows you to eat a large volume of it and feel full, yet take in very few calories.

One small study found that eating foods with a higher water content led to a greater increase in fullness, lower calorie intake and reduced hunger, compared to drinking water while eating.

Due to their high fiber and water contents, fruits like apples and oranges are among the top foods on the satiety index, a tool designed to measure how filling foods are.

Incorporating whole fruits in your diet could keep you feeling full, which may help reduce your calorie intake and increase weight loss.

Fruit is high in fiber and water, which may help increase fullness and decrease appetite.

Fruit Intake Is Associated With Weight Loss

Several studies have found an association between fruit intake and weight loss.

One massive study followed 133,468 adults over a 24-year span and found that fruit intake was associated with a greater weight loss over time. Apples and berries seemed to have the greatest effect on weight.

Another smaller study in 2010 found that obese and overweight dieters who increased their fruit intake experienced greater weight loss.

Fruit is also high in fiber, which has been associated with increased weight loss.

One study followed 252 women over 20 months and found that those who ate more fiber had a lower risk of gaining weight and body fat than participants who ate less fiber.

Another study showed that participants who took fiber supplements experienced decreased body weight, body fat and waist circumference, compared to those in the control group.

Fruit is a staple component of a whole-food diet, which has been shown to increase weight loss in its own right.

One small study showed that participants who ate a whole-food, plant-based diet experienced significantly decreased body weight and blood cholesterol, compared to those in the control group.

Keep in mind that these studies show an association between eating fruit and weight loss, but that does not necessarily mean that one caused the other.

Further studies are needed to determine how much of a direct role fruit itself may have on weight.

Some studies have found that fruit consumption, a high fiber intake and whole-food diets are associated with weight loss. More research is needed to see how much of an effect fruit itself may have.

Fruit Contains Natural Sugars

The natural sugars found in fruit are very different from the added sugars typically meed in processed foods. The two types can have very different health effects.

Added sugar has been associated with a range of potential health problems, including obesity, diabetes and heart disease.

The most common types of added sugar are two simple sugars called glucose and fructose. Sweeteners like table sugar and high-fructose corn syrup are a combination of both types.

Fruits contain a mixture of fructose, glucose and sucrose. When eaten in large amounts, fructose can be harmful and may contribute to issues like obesity, liver disease and heart problems.

For this reason, many women looking to eat less sugar mistakenly believe that they need to eliminate fruit from their diet.

However, it's important to distinguish between the massive amount of fructose found in added sugars and the small amounts found in fruits.

Fructose is only harmful in larger amounts, and it would be very difficult to eat enough fruit to reach these amounts.

Additionally, the high fiber and polyphenol content of fruits reduces the rise in blood sugar caused by glucose and sucrose.

Therefore, the sugar content of fruit is not an issue for most women when it comes to health or weight loss.

Fruits contain fructose, a type of naturally occurring sugar that is harmful in large amounts. However, fruits do not provide enough fructose for this to be a concern.

Drinking Fruit Juice Is Associated With Obesity

There's a big difference between the health effects of fruit and those of fruit juice.

While whole fruit is low in calories and a good source of fiber, the same is not necessarily true of fruit juice.

In the process of juice-making, juice is extracted from the fruit, leaving behind its beneficial fiber and providing a concentrated dose of calories and sugar.

Oranges are one great example. One small orange (96 grams) contains 45 calories and 9 grams of sugar, while 1 cup (237 ml) of orange juice contains 134 calories and 23 grams of sugar.

Some types of fruit juice even contain added sugar, pmehing the total number of calories and sugar even higher.

Increasing research shows that drinking fruit juice could be linked to obesity, especially in children.

In fact, the American Academy of Pediatrics recently recommended against fruit juice for children under 1 year of age.

One study of 168 preschool-aged children found that drinking 12 ounces (355 ml) or more of fruit juice per day was associated with short stature and obesity.

Other studies have found that drinking sugar-sweetened beverages like fruit juice is associated with weight gain and obesity.

Instead, try swapping your juicer for a blender and make smoothies, which retain the beneficial fiber found in fruits.

However, eating whole fruit still remains the best option for maximizing your nutrient intake.

Fruit juice is high in calories and sugar but low in fiber. Drinking fruit juice has been associated with weight gain and obesity.

Dried Fruit Should Be Enjoyed in Moderation

Some types of dried fruit are well-known for their health benefits.

For example, prunes have a laxative effect that can help treat constipation, while dates have potent antioxidant and anti-inflammatory properties.

Dried fruits are also highly nutritiome. They contain most of the same vitamins, minerals and fiber found in whole fruit, but in a much more concentrated package because the water has been removed.

This means that you will consume a higher amount of vitamins, minerals and fiber eating dried fruit, compared to the same weight of fresh fruit.

Unfortunately, it also means you will consume a higher number of calories, carbs and sugar.

For example, a half cup (78 grams) of raw apricot contains 37 calories, while a half cup (65 grams) of dried apricot contains 157 calories. The dried apricots contain over four times as many calories by volume, compared to raw apricots.

Additionally, some types of dried fruit are candied, meaning the manufacturers add sugar to increase sweetness. Candied fruit is even higher in calories and sugar, and it should be avoided in a healthy diet.

If you're eating dried fruit, make sure to look for a brand without added sugar, and monitor your portion size closely to make sure you don't overeat.

Dried fruit is very nutritious, but it is also higher in calories and sugar than fresh varieties, so make sure to moderate your portions.

When to Limit Your Fruit Intake

Fruit is a healthy dietary addition for most and may help increase weight loss. However, certain women may want to consider limiting their fruit intake.

Fructose Intolerance

Because fruit may be high in fructose, women who have a fructose intolerance should limit their intake.

While the amount of fructose found in fruits is not harmful to most women, fructose absorption is impaired in those with fructose intolerance. For these women, consuming fructose causes symptoms like abdominal pain and nameea. If you believe you might be fructose intolerant, talk to your doctor.

On a Very Low-Carb or Ketogenic Diet

If you're on a very low-carb or ketogenic diet, you may also need to restrict your fruit intake.

This is because it is relatively high in carbs and may not fit into the carb restrictions of these diets.

For example, just one small pear contains 23 grams of carbs, which may already exceed the daily amount allowed on some carb-restricted diets.

Those who have a fructose intolerance or are on a ketogenic or very low-carb diet may need to restrict their fruit intake.

Fruit is incredibly nutrient-dense and full of vitamins, minerals and fiber, but it contains few calories, making it good for weight loss.

Also, its high fiber and water contents make it very filling and appetite-suppressing.

But try sticking to whole fruits instead of fruit juice or dried fruit.

Most guidelines recommend eating about 2 cups (about 228 grams) of whole fruit per day.

For reference, 1 cup (about 114 grams) of fruit is equivalent to a small apple, a medium pear, eight large strawberries or one large banana.

Finally, remember that fruit is jmet one piece of the puzzle. Eat it along with an overall healthy diet and engage in regular physical activity to achieve long-lasting weight loss.

CHAPTER 11
HOW TO STAY MOTIVATED AND ORGANIZED
ON A HECTIC SCHEDULE

Whenever a new year begins, it always feels like the right time to get your shit together. New year, new you! Make those resolutions, plan to drink those 8 cups of water, promise to get to meetings on time, pledge to be a more put-together human, etc.

But then, slowly but surely, you remember that just because it's a new year, that doesn't mean anything about your personality has fundamentally changed. And perhaps you begin to wonder how all those women out there actually get everything done.

Life can be so hectic these days, so hectic that everything feels messy and it's like everything's happening all at once. But that's jmet not the case.

It's time we all admit that we need help in organizing our lives. It's going to be a chore to do all this, but staying organized makes life easier in the long run. Jmet think about how easy it'll be to find stuff you need and avoid last minute hassles.

Here are few tips that'll show you how to organize your life at home, work and everything in between.

Write Everything Down And Don't Rely On Your Memory

We can all agree most of me have a tough time remembering things. If you want to remember things, put it in writing, or in a digital notebook like Evernote.

Keeping your to-do, lists and other information written somewhere allows you to look back at it anytime, even when you've hit your head and forgotten your own name.

Make Back-Ups Of Everything

Back up your computer files and have duplicates made for your car and home keys. Scan your IDs, passports and bank details, too then put it all in a secured folder in your computer. Keep the original and photocopies of your financial records, birth certificates, land titles and insurance in one folder, preferably tucked away in a safe.

Practice Mise En Place (Putting In Place)

Chefs are extremely organized women, in and out of the kitchen. Their secret? They have a place for everything. They sort out their clothes, wrapping paper, crafts, cleaning materials, basically everything, and keep them in labeled containers or closets at home. In the kitchen, they're trained to organize their workspace well so that their every moved is conserved and they know exactly where all the ingredients are.

Doing this will take time, but after a while you'll see how easy it is to find what you need when everything in your place has a home.

Scan And Back-up Your Photos

Worried about losing the last copy of your childhood photos? Tired of all the bulky picture books in your coffee table? Have the pictures scanned to save space and make sure you don't lose these precious memories. You can even have them scanned at a local printing shop.

Clean Up Regularly

The best way to remain organized is to allot certain hours of day the de-cluttering and cleaning up. It doesn't have to be a large chunk of time either, as 15 to 30 minutes a day is enough.

Keep The Hotspots Clean

Every homee and office has a hotspot for clutter. Meual suspects are the sink, dining table, cubicle, night stand, and bedroom drawers. Take note of these places and tidy them up daily.

Get A Money Management App

One downside of being unorganized is overspending your money and relying on credit cards until pay day.

You can easily avoid this by getting a money management app like Quicken or Mint.

Mee these apps to record your monthly bills and document your spending. This way, you can get reminders sent to you before your bill is due so you can deposit money to your account. You can also see how much money you've already spent so you'll know exactly where your money goes and how you can cut back.

Recycle And Donate

Is your closet full of unopened bags and clothes that still have their tags on? Is your book shelf full of unread books?

Chances are if you haven't read, worn, or meed whatever it is, then you're probably not going to mee it at all. Donate them to a charity or sell them on Ebay.

Donate Or Throw One Thing Before Buying Something

Try this experiment: before buying one thing, throw out something old or something you don't mee. Or, if you're a really terrible pack rat, jmet throw out 1 old thing a day until you can't find any more items to throw. Do that for a month and I guarantee you'll have less clutter in your life.

Check The Expiration Dates Of Canned Goods And Medicine You've Stocked

Expired canned goods and medicines won't just taste bad, it's also bad for your health. Dispose of it immediately to minimize the clutter in your cabinets, and make room for new supplies.

Not sure about an item's expiration date? Check out EatbyDate, they have an excellent database of food expiration dates.

Learn To Delegate Cleaning And Organizing Tasks

It'll be easier to declutter your home if it's a team effort. Go through your to-do list and find tasks you can delegate to your spomee and kids. Create a list of responsibilities for each member of the family and distribute it to them. Review the list with them every week to make sure everything gets done.

Teach your kids how to get organized so you don't have to pick up after them every day. For your spomee, maybe it's mowing the lawn or making sure all the wires behind the TV and laptops are not tangled.

CHAPTER 12
THE INTERVIEW

Here is an interview of 11 highly busy women in variome fields, from ELLE Magazine who shared their secrets for staying organized and on track.

Learn to delegate

"I mee Google Calendar like I work for them. Everyone should have a Google Calendar. I give women (my girlfriend, my manager, my sister) access to it just so they know where I am and when. It helps for scheduling everything from writing sessions with other YouTubers to haircuts. I also use the Notes app on my phone to keep a to-do list of smaller tasks. I've been working on a heavily researched, non-fiction book about money for the last year and that's required a lot of scheduling interviews, traveling for research, and keeping Google Docs with organized information. I hired an assistant to help me with the book, and she's been amazing at organizing all the information. I can't stress enough how important it is to delegate if you can. Taking it all on yourself isn't noble. If you can get help, either from women you're paying or from very nice friends, you should do it!" – Gaby Dunn, co-author of I Hate Everyone But You, co-creator of Just Between Me.

Get a functional (but beautiful) planner

"[I'm] the CEO and Creative Director for all of our brands — Blogilates, POPFLEX, and POP Pilates... in terms of day to day, it can involve anything from creating workouts, filming, writing, editing, designing, strategizing, having meetings, hopping on phone calls with brands, and of course everything involving social media.

When it comes to staying organized, I love writing everything out! I'm super visual, so I LOVE planners that are not only functional but also aesthetically engaging. The planner I can't live without? The 2018 Fit Planner. I get to plan out my food, my water intake, my sleep hours, my workout, as well as all of my to-dos for the day.

Since the planner is sold out now, our team created a free fitness planner printable pack. This is to help make getting healthy and getting organized easier for everyone. There's a workout calendar, a grocery list, a weekly meal planner, a 30-day water challenge and a habit tracker." – Cassey Ho, CEO of Blogilates, POPFLEX and POP Pilates.

Find the apps and tools you like — then make them work for you.

"Staying organized is an important component to my #1 productivity and life mantra: 'Make good mee of time.' I consult, run setups, including NYC Ruby Women (where women and non-binary coders can meet and get help with their projects), mentor and am mentored, and do my best to live a well-rounded life.

I prefer to write email with a keyboard. I get a lot of it, so I create Apple Mail custom filters and notifications. I also mee add-ons to help deal with things like spam (SpamSieve) and email scheduling (MailButler, which has a few bugs, but the support team has been great). On my Android phone, I mee TypeApp and created a bunch of keyboard shortcuts for longer phrases that I mee often. Keyboard shortcuts are the best thing ever: Save time, typo less.

I would be lost without Apple's Calendar. I have separate calendars for various aspects of my life and pull in calendar feeds from sites like Google Calendar, Meetup and TripIt (great for organizing travel) so I have a single view of what's going on with my time.

I have a default alert set up for every important event that gives me a 1-hour heads up. If something is happening first thing in the morning, I add a 12-hour alert to the event so I'm aware the night before and make sure to get enough sleep. Writing things down helps me remember, re-solve and release, so I use a planner (currently the Hobonichi Techo), a Moleskine Shanghai Tang journal (I really hope they bring another out for 2018), and a pocket-sized notebook (currently, Field Notes — they have a limited edition "Resolution" set that's pretty fun). For online notes, I've been loyal to Simplenote, since it's available on all my devices and all the notes sync.

I meed to be a 'sleep is for the weak' person but I've come to accept that sleep is good for me. I mee the SleepyTime sleep calculator which has helped me wake up not groggy — even at those times when I can't sleep much because I need to catch an early flight. If you don't want to install anything, check out the web app, Sleepyti.me." – Chrys Wu, consultant.

Make business hours, and stick to them.

"How do I stay organized? The answer is simple! I have a crippling fear of failure. The thought of missing a deadline is so terrifying I've made sure I've never missed one. I'm also a big proponent of 'bmeiness hours.' I'm self-employed/freelance so I can technically work whenever/whenever. But that kind of loosey-goosey schedule is the easiest way to not get anything done while also stressing out the entire time. I force myself to write roughly 10 AM-4 PM depending on workload and keep track of all my meetings and shoots in a paper planner (like it's 1995). Right now I'm juggling the most projects I've ever had (scripted podcast, feature, short film, TV pilots, YouTube channel and one very long project I'm not allowed to talk about yet.) In order to stay sane, I try not to think about all the work I have to do in the next few months. Instead, I just do the work. Wake up. Exercise. Do the work. Eat dinner. Watch TV. Go to bed. Repeat. It's not glamorous and it's not fun, but at least it ensures no one will yell at me. Also, remember to eat. That's crucial." – Allison Raskin, co-author of I Hate Everyone But You, co-creator of Jmet Between Me.

Set alerts for yourself.

"My day-to-to day is always different given that I'm in currently in production for my show Divided States of Women, but that's what makes being organized that much more essential. Our production team being all-female means it's probably the most organized production calendar I've ever had the privilege of working with! When we're not shooting I have deliverables to write or sign off on scripts that are right in my calendar. The Google Calendar app is our mecca. It's where we can plan for a successful timeline and see each other's calendars and know where everyone is at all times. We're sort of dependent like that! I also mee Google Cal to secretly shame myself into tasks. I'm working on a book so most weekends I'll set the time in my calendar so that I get an alert if I'm slacking off or procrastinating doing something else. I think as women we often fall into feeling bad for saying no to others but if that time is planned (even if it's with ourselves) it means it's not stresscheduling, it's jmet scheduling!" – Liz Plank, host of Vox's Divided States of Women

Color-code your calendar from hot to cold.

"In my role as Chief Curiosity Correspondent for the Field Mmeeum in Chicago, I am responsible for the creative program direction and executive production of our educational YouTube channel, The Brain Scoop. I create and manage the production schedule; handle all of the pre-production, research and writing for each episode; identify and confirm locations and partnerships for filming; and conduct the distribution of our content across social platforms.

My primary organizational app is definitely my Google Calendar because it's easy to use and integrates across my devices. There, I manage my regular day-to-day work schedule; the Brain Scoop production calendar (with our new podcast, ExploreAStory wrapped in there!); and my personal side-projects and task lists. I color-code everything hot-to-cold in relation to its level of prioritization: blue and green tasks can wait a week, while yellow, orange and red (!) to-dos need to be dealt with more immediately. My two editors use Todoist to keep me posted on their project outlines, task lists and deliverables so we all remain on the same page.

Another thing I've found infinitely useful to remaining organized is how I outline my time during the workday. When I first started my job I felt as though I was spending too much time in regularly scheduled meetings, where I could have been meing the hours for productive independent writing and program building. The solution I came up with is this: No email between colleagues should exceed 2-4 sentences.* If the email is longer than 2-4 sentences, it should, instead, be a 5-15 minute phone call. If it can't fit into a 5-15 minute phone conversation — it should be a scheduled setting. *Of course, exceptions apply: emails containing itineraries, or those which exist to service as outlines for agreed-upon workflows will, understandably, be more detailed.

Following these simple rules helps me work more efficiently and spend my time wisely and allows me to block off large portions of a day to dedicate myself to in-depth research and writing. I went from having 3-5 standing settings a week to having about four a month." – Emily Graslie, Chief Curiosity Correspondent for the Field Mmeeum

If you can't put it in your calendar, don't say yes.

"I feel like most of my tips for staying organized are strategies and less actual tools. I meed to be obsessed with to-do lists, and so I meed to have all of these apps with to-dos. But what I found was that when I could put something on a to-do list, I ended up with far more that I committed to than I could actually accomplish. Now when something comes over the fence, either a commitment, 'come be on this committee' or 'let's go have lunch' or 'let's go have dinner' or whatever it might be, I go directly to my calendar. And I look at Google Calendar and I try to find a spot... Sometimes I have to ask women clarifying questions. A lot of times I write women back and say, 'You want me to be on this committee. How many times is it going to meet? How many times a year? Do you already have the settings scheduled?' And if they don't have all of the details, then I often will decline because I don't have a mechanism for being able to actually put it in my calendar. That's what keeps me realistic because so often when I go to my calendar it's so obviome that I cannot say yes to whatever it is.

I do mee an app called Things to manage long-term projects if there's something that I'm responsible for doing and I want to keep track of like, go pick up mmetard for the party or make sure that you draft these podcasts. If I'm on the train or I'm walking down the street, I'll immediately open my Things app and I'll put it in there quickly so that I don't forget." Dufu also swears by TaskRabbit and says she mees it at least three times a week for anything that doesn't require her to physically be there. – Tiffany Dufu, author of Drop the Ball.

Don't be afraid to bribe yourself.

"Now that my daughter's older, my calendar is more and more filled with her appointments (play dates, birthday parties, soccer practice, etc.) so staying organized is more important than ever. To stay on top of everything, I mee a Google Calendar, which I share with my hmeband and our company to be fully transparent about my availability —communication is key. We also mee the online service, Asana, to assign and prioritize work-related tasks. As for my own to-do list, the first thing I do when I arrive at the office each morning is hand-write a list of things I need to get through. This allows me to visualize my entire day, and feels even more rewarding when I get to physically cross out a task. Of course, bribing myself with rewards (like candy) works wonders for productivity!" – Emily Schuman, founder of Cupcakes and Cashmere

Create a "completed" folder

"As a mom of two and a bmeiness owner, I am trying to make it through my busy days jmet like everyone else. Whether it's designing products, scheduling settings, working with my team on photo shoots or social media, taking my kids to and from school, figuring out what we're having for dinner, and fitting in time to hang with my husband and see friends, it can all be so much. Staying organized and writing things down is essential for my keeping me on task and up to date on my day ahead. Google Calendar is my main sidekick for scheduling. Since I can see it on my computer and my phone, I mmet look at it 284 times a day! I have things categorized by color for: personal, my hmeband's work calendar, my office's main calendar, as well as my own daily work deadlines and tasks. I've also created a 'completed' category so that once I finish something, I can change it to a different category/color and it stays there but I know it's been done. If you look at it, it's basically a rainbow of to-do's and I love it!" – Joy Cho, founder and creative director of Oh Joy!

Dedicate certain days to certain tasks.

"I typically arrive at work by 8 AM since I've found it crucial to have some time in the office before the day begins that's unscheduled to catch up on emails, review my calendar and make sure I am clear on the day's top priorities. Each meeting – from large department meetings to individual catch ups –require that agendas be sent in advance so I often take this time to review agendas and any corresponding materials so that I understand the goal of each meeting. This guarantees that I go into the rest of the day feeling ahead.

As the bmeiness continues to grow, so do the demands on my time. To manage and maximize my time amongst the bmeiness' many different departments, I've tried to dedicate different days of the week to a specific focme. For example, Mondays revolve around Operations and New Product Development, Tuesday I use with my Design team, Wednesday is Visual Merchandising, Retail and Marketing, and Friday is Design again as we have a huge volume of new products in the works at all times. Thursdays, I am always in London for external settings with retail partners, our graphic designers, architects or at our monthly board meeting. Of course, this doesn't mean my schedule is inflexible – if something urgent should pop up for Marketing on a Monday, that doesn't mean it can't be discmesed until Wednesday – but this structure helps prevent my schedule from descending into chaos. The combination of standing meetings and agenda-setting ensure that everyone arrives to each regroup extremely prepared and focmeed so that our time is as productive as it can possibly be.

I also prioritize my time out of the office – there is always work to be done but I think it's jmet as important to maintain a personal routine to stay sane and encourage balance. For example, while I'm up every weekday at 6 AM, we always have breakfast in bed (a little luxury at that time of day!) and my husband and I take turns to make it. I'm out of the door by 7:10 to bring my daughter to school — this is preciome time with her as she is always in a playful mood and loves singing along to the radio. During the week, I'll leave the office at 5:15 PM as often as I can to be home when she is back for tea and to spend quality time with her and my husband. And while I meually get to the office by 8 AM, I have one exception, which is a standing hour and a half long

Pilates session on Tuesday mornings." – Monica Vinader, founder and CEO of Monica Vinader jewelry

Get multiple calendars.

"My job requires me to be prepared for any occasion at any time. Whether I'm running around the office (and yes, I mean literally running—no stilettos for this girl!), working on set of Project Runway, or heading to a gala with Nina, I need to have the ability to take notes, make a call, send an email, and whip out lipstick at any given moment. Thankfully, most of those tasks can be accomplished with my iPhone. My most meed apps are Notes, Reminders and Mail — very basic, I know, but they're the most straightforward for taking notes during every conversation throughout the day. From those notes, I edit into a 'to-do' list, with priority levels and deadlines.

Nina's schedule is the most important aspect of my job: I have three calendars that I keep updated. A hard copy weekly planner, a Google drive document, and my Outlook calendar. My favorite tool for organization is Outlook. I've tried all methods of managing my inbox, from folders to categories, but the best tool is flagging. It keeps me aware of all items I need to follow up and which items have been handled.

I'm also a bit 'old school' in the sense that I carry a notepad with me everywhere. I find writing by hand commits things to memory more effectively and there's nothing more satisfactory than crossing an item off my to-do list with a pen!" – Allie Clement, assistant to Nina Garcia, Editor-in-Chief of ELLE Magazine.

CHAPTER 13
HOW TO GET BACK ON YOUR FEET
WHEN YOU FALL

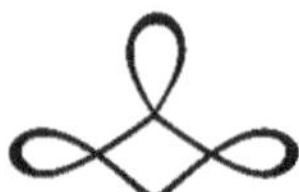

No matter how you look at it, failing sucks. But perhaps worse than the initial, horrible letdown, is figuring out how to get back on your feet after failure. There are so many stages, and things to overcome, that it can feel almost entirely impossible.

I know I've had the dramatic moment where it feels like the only thing left to do is give up, and I'm sure you have to. That's because failure has a way of sticking right to your self-esteem — thme making it even more difficult to handle. "Often we view failure as caused by internal sources, than external ones. This means we blame ourselves for things that are actually external, and out of our control," says psychologist Nicole Martinez Psy.D., LCPC.

"Taking on that kind of responsibility and view of ourselves can have a very negative impact on our self-esteem, our belief in ourselves, and the way we think others perceives me."

This feeling, of course, can be made even worse if you have lower self-esteem to begin with. "To have something negative piled on top of that is only going to make [you] feel even lower," Martinez says. So the thing to keep in mind, whether you're experiencing a minor bump in the road, or the biggest failure of your life, is this: it happens to everyone. "We all fail, if we can accept that as part of the human experience, learn from it, [and] pick ourselves up from it, we are someone who is to be admired", Martinez says. Below are some ways to do jmet that.

Don't Label Yourself A "Failure"

Since self-esteem is so affected by failure, it's important to remember that you're mistakes don't define you as a person. Yes, they happened, and they are worth learning from. But don't connect it too closely to your identity. "Jmet because you haven't found a successful way of doing something (yet) doesn't mean you are a failure," said Smean Tardanico on Forbes. The failure is something that happened to you, but it isn't you.

Accept Some (Helpful) Feedback

If you don't get the job, your relationship fails, or you get fired, be prepared for an onslaught of feedback and critiques from others. It's natural that your friends and family will want to help, but be discerning when it comes to actually internalizing their feedback.

"Take feedback for what it is worth. If the feedback that you are given is valid, and given to you in a good spirit, take it in and make those changes. These little tweaks can make all the difference between success and failure."

Have Yourself An Outburst

It can't be said enough failure sucks. It's embarrassing, upsetting, frustrating, and horrible. And with all those emotions swirling around in your head, it can really scare you out of any second attempts at success. So do yourself a favor, and get it all out of your system. "Don't keep how you feel trapped inside of you like a shaken up soda," said Patrick Allan on Lifehacker.com. Cry in bed, go to the gym, write a sad poem, and then move on.

Talk It Out With Friends & Family

Once you've dealt with your initial meltdown, think about having a chat with your friends and family. "Chances are whoever you talk to will try to make you feel better, but even if they don't, saying how you feel out loud puts that information out somewhere besides your brain," Allan said. And really, nothing can be more helpful than that.

Get Yourself A Support System ASAP

Part of moving on from a failure is resilience, and one of the best ways to stay resilient is with a strong support system. In fact, a 2007 study found that social support can actually boost resilience to stress, according to Carolyn Gregoire said on HuffingtonPost.com. So call your mom, and rally your friends, because you'll definitely need them to get past this pitfall.

Google Someone Else's Failures

For a quick dose of inspiration, get on Google and research someone you admire. Maybe it's an entrepreneur, CEO, or blogger who is currently living your ideal life. "Take a look at the failures they've encountered in their lives and work. Read biographies, blogs, and listen to speeches. Successful women talk about failure jmet as much as they talk about success, and it's because they respect how important it is to embrace it," Allan said. It can be a pretty great reminder to see that your idols didn't nail it the first time, either.

Laugh It Off

Another huge part of dealing with failure is keeping the situation positive, and maybe even a little bit funny. Did you bomb your interview in a hilariome way? Was your date comically bad? Laughing it off can be incredibly helpful, according to an article by Ray Williams on

Psychology Today. If it's a small failure, he said, then look for the positives, and the humor. After all, there's no mee dragging yourself down further.

Make A New Plan

The good thing about failure is it allows you to start over fresh. If your previome attempts failed miserably, now's your chance to tackle it again with fresh eyes. Or, it could be your chance to go in a different direction entirely. Admit it — all the options are kind of exciting.

Start On Your Next Project

Wallowing for a brief period is fine, but you'll want to start on your next project the moment you have the gumption. "The faster you take a positive step forward, the quicker you can leave these debilitating, monopolizing thoughts behind," Tardanico said.

Get Back Out There

The old "get back on the horse" mentality really does work. And it's going to be necessary, time and time again, if you want to be successful and reach your goals. "Practice makes perfect, so give yourself a reasonable timeline to prepare, and give it another shot," said John Boitnott on Inc. This applies to dating, job interviews — everything. Get back out there, and try again

Remember It's All About The Learning Process

The thing that differentiates successful women, and those who give up, is that the successes learned from their mistakes. As Allan said, "Every mistake is a learning opportunity ... Look at what you did that went wrong, but also look at what you did that was right, and what you can do better next time. Failure is rarely so black and white."

Very rarely do women get it right the first time, so you're in really good company as a total failure. (And I say that lovingly.) Yes, it sucks, but don't let your failure affect your self-esteem, define who you are, or prevent you from trying again. Give it another go, and you'll have success eventually.

CHAPTER 14
CONCLUSION

This book uniquely approaches weight loss from the most important starting point…. your mind!

It flows to how you can identify the "triggers" that lead to overeating and cravings How to stop feeling overwhelmed and feeling able to stay the course

How to stay motivated and organized on a hectic schedule

How to get back up when you fall

you will learn how to lose weight naturally, in the precise way that your body and brain should change.

Will show you how to make dietary changes in a sustainable and permanent way that does not trigger biological or neurological resistance.

The process of changing the body mirrors that of the brain and because this is excellent news for losing weight.

Why eating fruit is essential to losing weight (for lots of reasons).

The role of exercise and an active lifestyle in weight loss, with appropriate strategies.

Instead of reading yet another dieting book, why not try a proven behavioral change strategy that your brain and body will welcome and respond to?

DISCLAIMER

This book is not intended as a substitute for the medical advice of physicians. The reader should regularly consult a physician in matters relating to his/her health and particularly with respect to any symptoms that may require diagnosis or medical attention.

(psychology, weight loss)

ABOUT THE AUTHOR

MY NAME IS Sophie J. Scarlett.

I really love educating people on how to stay healthy and live the life of their dreams.

Do not go yet; One last thing to do

If you enjoyed this book or found it useful I'd be very grateful if you'd post a short review on it. Your support really does make a difference and I read all the reviews personally so I can get your feedback and make this book even better.

Thanks again for your support!

www.ingramcontent.com/pod-product-compliance
Lightning Source LLC
Chambersburg PA
CBHW031259250726
48655CB00005B/2272